Headline Series

No. 290   **FOREIGN POLICY ASSOCIATION**   Fall 1989

The Cocaine Connection

Drug Trafficking and Inter-American Relations

by Merrill Collett

Cover Design: Ed Bohon $4.00

HV
5810
.C6
1989

The Author

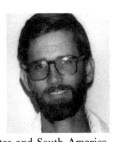

MERRILL COLLETT is an award-winning, free-lance foreign correspondent who covers the Andean region from his base in Venezuela, where he has lived since 1984. He has written on the drug issue for *The Nation*, *Newsweek*, *The Washington Post*, *The Christian Science Monitor*, *The New Statesman* and *The Columbia Journalism Review*, and his articles and reports on Latin America have been carried by more than 40 newspapers, magazines, news services, newsletters and radio news shows in Europe, Canada, the United States and South America.

He has degrees from Stanford University and Johns Hopkins University, and he studied Latin American affairs at Cornell University on a National Defense Foreign Language Fellowship. In May 1988 he received a grant from The Fund for Investigative Journalism to study the relationship between cocaine traffickers and Peru's Maoist guerrillas.

The Foreign Policy Association

The Foreign Policy Association is a private, nonprofit, nonpartisan educational organization. Its purpose is to stimulate wider interest and more effective participation in, and greater understanding of, world affairs among American citizens. Among its activities is the continuous publication, dating from 1935, of the HEADLINE SERIES. The author is responsible for factual accuracy and for the views expressed. FPA itself takes no position on issues of U.S. foreign policy.

HEADLINE SERIES (ISSN 0017-8780) is published four times a year, Winter, Spring, Summer and Fall, by the Foreign Policy Association, Inc., 729 Seventh Ave., New York, N.Y. 10019. Chairman, Robert V. Lindsay; President, John W. Kiermaier; Editor in Chief, Nancy L. Hoepli; Senior Editors, Ann R. Monjo and K.M. Rohan. Subscription rates, $15.00 for 4 issues; $25.00 for 8 issues; $30.00 for 12 issues. Single copy price $4.00. Discount 25% on 10 to 99 copies; 30% on 100 to 499; 35% on 500 to 999; 40% on 1,000 or more. Payment must accompany all orders. Add $1.75 for postage. USPS #238-340. Second-class postage paid at New York, N.Y. POSTMASTER: Send address changes to HEADLINE SERIES, Foreign Policy Association, 729 Seventh Ave., New York, N.Y. 10019. Copyright 1989 by Merrill Collett. Composed and printed at Science Press, Ephrata, Pennsylvania. Fall 1989.

Library of Congress Catalog Card No. 89-85130
ISBN 0-87124-128-5

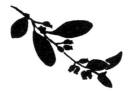

Introduction

According to a story told on the Caribbean coast of Colombia, a U.S. sailor came ashore one day and asked a boy on the beach to bring him some marijuana. When the boy returned with a bagful, the sailor asked the price. Fifty, said the boy. He meant 50 Colombian pesos, but the sailor misunderstood and paid 50 U.S. dollars, an enormously larger sum. At that moment the illegal drug business was born, or so the story goes.

The apocryphal tale contains a core of truth. The high prices U.S. citizens paid for marijuana and cocaine stimulated Latin Americans and other growers to supply these drugs. It took both halves of the Western Hemisphere to make the inter-American drug trade what it is today—a vast industry that unites consumers in the United States with producers in Latin America.

Until very recently the United States did not acknowledge that it was one half of the drug-trade equation. Although U.S. citizens freely imported and used narcotics, the United States saw itself besieged by Latin American traffickers and invaded by their nefarious products. U.S. government officials played up the foreign origin of drugs while giving little importance to the fact that many if not most drug users were native born. This one-sided perspective skewed the focus of U.S. antidrug action. Having decided that the source of the drug problem was overseas, Washington ordered its drug fighters to "go to the source." Thus most of the big battles in the U.S. war on drugs have been fought on Latin American soil.

The Latin View

The assumption that drug trafficking was primarily a Latin American problem was never shared by the Latins themselves. When the United States blamed foreign drug suppliers, Latin leaders blamed U.S. drug consumers. "Colombians are not corrupting Americans. You are corrupting us. If you abandon illegal drugs, the traffic will disappear," Colombian President Julio César Turbay Ayala said 10 years ago. In 1988 Washington started listening closely to what the Latin Americans were saying. After steadily losing ground to foreign traffickers, the Reagan Administration shifted its drug-fighting focus to the domestic front with a "zero-tolerance" program that promised to "get the users and prosecute them, no matter how small the quantity of the illegal drug found in their possession."

It remains to be seen whether or not the repression of drug use at home will be more successful than attempts to suppress trafficking abroad, but at least the United States has moved away from blaming its drug habits on its southern neighbors. The way is cleared for the new Administration of President George Bush to carry out a drug policy that sees the Latin American countries as allies against the traffickers, not their accomplices.

The necessity to unite against the drug traffickers raises the possibility that the United States and Latin America will achieve new levels of cooperation on other mutual problems, such as foreign debt, immigration and the preservation of the ecology. If the danger of drugs serves to strengthen hemispheric coordination, it will have produced something good in the long run. In the short run, however, drugs are a threat that must be confronted. Will the United States fall back on the failed policies of the past? Or can it forge its mistakes into an effective antidrug program? At a time when U.S. drug policy stands at the crossroads, this HEADLINE SERIES looks back at where the United States has been and attempts to shed some light on where it should go.

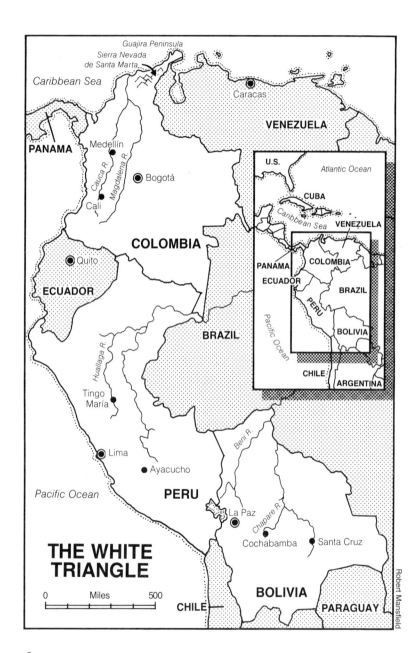

THE WHITE TRIANGLE

0   Miles   500

Robert Mansfield

1

Evolution of an Industry

Over the last decade drug trafficking has established itself as the world's fastest-growing industry, and business is getting better. Despite some evidence that the consumption of marijuana and cocaine is leveling off in the United States, U.S. citizens still spend an estimated $100 billion per year on illegal narcotics, and the European demand for drugs is rising. The amount of land dedicated to the cultivation of drug-producing plants increases every year. Smuggling rings have grown from crime syndicates into vertically integrated conglomerates. More and more nations are being drawn into the drug-supply network, either as producers or as transit routes. How did this happen?

The new industry grew out of a U.S. social revolution in the 1960s that stripped away the social stigma associated with drug use. Marijuana became fashionable among young North Americans. When they started buying marijuana in Mexican border towns, neighbors to the south heard opportunity knock. The cultivation of marijuana earned Mexican peasants many times more than any other crop, and soon the tall, green plants were sprouting on the western slopes of the Sierra Madre and truckloads of "pot" were heading north to the booming U.S.

market. In 1964 U.S. Customs Service agents confiscated 7,000 pounds of marijuana, mostly at the Mexican border. Experts believe that for many years the interdiction of marijuana only netted 3 percent of the amount actually smuggled in, which means that even at this early date the United States imported 100 metric tons of the drug in a single year.

Mexicans supplied most of the U.S. demand for marijuana in the 1960s, but in the early 1970s the United States pressured the Mexican government to begin spraying the herbicide paraquat on marijuana fields. U.S. pot smokers had to turn to other sources. Jamaica was one of them, and the fledgling domestic U.S. industry was another, but it was Colombia that filled the vacuum left by the collapse of Mexican supply. By the end of the decade Colombia provided nearly three quarters of the marijuana smuggled into the United States.

Colombians entered into the trade with their own variety of the cannabis plant. Grown in the fertile coastal mountains of the Sierra Nevada de Santa Marta, "Colombian Gold" had a distinctive yellow color and a strong potency that made it the drug of choice for pot smokers who could afford to pay its higher price. But the Colombians were not content with a small share of the booming U.S. market. Demonstrating a capacity for inventive entrepreneurship that would characterize the Colombian cocaine smugglers who were to follow, the marijuana traffickers adopted a new mode of transport that allowed them to expand greatly the volume of marijuana shipped. They loaded it onto freighters and fishing trawlers and carried it to the Eastern Seaboard of the United States. There they rendezvoused with small boats that delivered the drugs to distributors on shore. In 1974 agents of the U.S. Drug Enforcement Administration (DEA) in New Orleans discovered 24 tons of marijuana on one of the mother ships.

Pot of Gold

Colombian involvement in the U.S. marijuana trade ended at the wholesale level and did not extend into street distribution, but with pot selling for at least $300 a pound wholesale and Americans consuming about 9,000 tons of the drug every year from all sources, according to conservative estimates, the Colombian traffickers earned fabulous profits nonetheless. How much they earned is a matter of informed speculation. A frequently seen number is $1 billion annually, but illicit drug business statistics are notoriously unreliable. Although it is a global industry, its companies publish no annual reports, and research very quickly becomes a matter of sorting out the best guesses. First there is the problem of obtaining information about an illegal activity deliberately obscured by those involved in it. Second, illegal narcotics is such a highly emotional issue that even objective analysts are subject to strong biases that skew their results. The problem is even more acute when it comes to data supplied by politicians and governments. As RAND Corporation economist Peter Reuter notes in his 1984 article in *The Public Interest,* officials often use the drug issue to build public support for their own agendas. Every statistic on drugs—prices, volume, earnings, arrests, numbers of users and addicts—must be interpreted in this light. But although drug statistics are imprecise, they can point toward reasonable generalizations. In the case of marijuana, the numbers suggest that the new industry had a major impact on Colombian coastal society.

Marijuana cultivation is highly labor intensive. One U.S. political scientist who has done interviews along the Caribbean coast of Colombia says that by the end of the 1970s the industry employed 30,000 to 50,000 peasants who lived entirely on the sale of their *marimba* (marijuana) crops and another 50,000 people who had some role in the trade, such as guards, drivers, seasonal laborers and bankers. The most conspicuous members of the drug business were those who ran it. Newly rich *marimberos* cruised about in luxury cars and built beach resorts where they could display their wealth, but not all of the *narcotraficantes* were nouveaux riches. Old, landed families on the coast, with roots reaching back to the Spanish conquest, were attracted by the easy money of the marijuana bonanza. Shielded by their inherited political influence, they built up networks of drug dealers and tapped into the new source of wealth. For the most part these members of Colombia's traditional oligarchy used their marijuana money to replenish failing family fortunes and firm up their social status. Once that was done, they retired from the trade, leaving behind a legacy of corrupted public officials and dead antidrug agents. Neither the old families nor the marimberos followed the drug business into its next, more profitable and more violent phase of cocaine trafficking. Today Colombia continues to export large amounts of marijuana to the United States, but its market share has been pushed down to about one quarter of the total by competition from domestic U.S. growers, by the resurgence of Mexican supply and by aggressive interdiction, since marijuana is bulky and thus easy to detect.

Cocaine—the Miracle Drug

Cocaine is derived from the shiny green leaves of a South American shrub known to botanists as *Erythroxylon* and to the Aymara Indians of the Andes as coca, a word that means simply plant or tree, suggesting that coca is so central to Indian culture that it is *the* plant. Writing in the January 1989 *National Geographic,* Peter T. White points out that the coca shrub has been cultivated by Indians for many millennia to be used as a folk medicine, a sacrament in their religious rituals and a mild stimulant that provides renewed energy and increased mental clarity, rather like a cup of coffee. Today the younger generation of Indians seems to be moving away from the practice of chewing coca, but there are millions who still wedge a wad of dried coca leaves into a corner of their mouths. The United Nations contends that coca leaf mastication harms mental processes, but that assessment is based on research that is nearly 40 years old. Most medical experts now say that coca is not physically damaging and may be of benefit by providing calories and vitamins for malnourished populations. Cocaine is another matter. When a German chemist isolated the active alkaloids in coca leaves, he converted a mild stimulant into a toxic drug.

The invention of cocaine is attributed to Friedrich Gaedcke, a German chemist who distilled a white crystalline powder from coca leaves in 1855. European doctors were soon singing the praises of the new miracle substance. They said it anesthetized the body without dulling the mind, and surgeons used it in eye and throat operations. Cocaine moved into mass consumption when a Corsican chemist and entrepreneur named Angelo Mariani patented a mixture of coca extract and wine. His "Vin Mariani" won the endorsements of Sarah Bernhardt, Thomas Edison and Pope Leo XIII and was a smash success in the United States. In 1885 a pharmacist in Georgia entered the booming U.S. market for cocaine products with Coca-Cola, which he sold first as a coca wine, then as a medicine and finally as "the intellectual beverage and temperance drink." The advertisements for these and the other proliferating cocaine-based drinks, syrups, balms and powders stressed their therapeutic benefit as a pick-me-up. Doctors generally supported the claim that these nostrums contributed to mental well-being, and in 1884 Sigmund Freud wrote an influential paper in praise of cocaine euphoria. Freud experimented with its use himself and administered it to his friends. One of them became painfully dependent on the drug, pointing the way toward the coming shift in medical opinion. By the end of the century, doctors were warning against the dangers of cocaine addiction. In 1906 the Pure Food and Drug Act required the listing of narcotic ingredients on labels of patent medicines, and the Harrison Narcotic Act of 1914 required that the production and sale of opiates and cocaine be registered and records kept. Cocaine declined in popularity throughout the 1920s, and by 1930 it had sunk into the North American underground as an illicit white powder that was sniffed by jazz musicians, movie stars and wealthy eccentrics.

The 1960s saw the birth of a rebellious youth movement whose slogan was "drugs, sex and rock and roll." Cocaine, whose harmful effects had been forgotten, emerged from the underground. It only gradually entered the mainstream of U.S. life, however. The 1960s subculture at first regarded cocaine as an expensive, inaccessible drug whose hard-edged euphoria could be achieved more cheaply and more easily with amphetamines. But by the end of the decade amphetamines were passing out of favor as a hazardous drug, and a police crackdown was making them more difficult to obtain. Encouraged by movies whose heroes were cocaine dealers (*Easy Rider, Superfly*), and by rock musicians, who had started wearing tiny "coke" spoons around their necks, young North Americans were attracted to the drug, whose high cost added to its glamour. Cocaine consumption started to rise. In 1970 the U.S. government seized 305 pounds of cocaine. The next year the volume more than doubled, to 787 pounds. Cocaine was taking off as a chic narcotic. In time it would move from the drug culture into middle-class culture, becoming a required luxury of the affluent. In 1985 U.S. agents seized over 50,000 pounds of the white powder.

Did pot smokers "graduate" to coke sniffing? There is evidence that marijuana traffickers in Miami, Florida, shifted to smuggling cocaine when the drug became popular, but there is nothing in the pharmacology of either drug to suggest that marijuana created a need for cocaine. Their effects are different: marijuana enervates while cocaine energizes. The link between the drugs is social, rather than physiological. The use of both has a common origin in the defiant subculture that encouraged youth to challenge social taboos against the use of narcotics. In the 1960s consumption increased for every illicit drug—heroin, LSD, Quaaludes, PCP, barbiturates, inhalants and others. Cocaine rose to popularity on this wave of mass experimentation.

Bolivian Pioneers

In 1970 Bolivia and Peru grew almost all of the world's coca. It was legally cultivated in these two countries to supply the internal demand for leaves and the foreign demand for soft-drink flavoring and pharmaceuticals. It was illegal to manufacture coca derivatives, but coca production started to turn in that direction as the news of the U.S. hunger for cocaine reached the Andes. The first to respond were agro-industrialists living in the Bolivian departments of Beni and Santa Cruz, remote rural regions which reached to the borders with Brazil and Paraguay and had a long tradition of smuggling. The landowners in the area were agile businessmen who had become wealthy by quickly shifting from one agricultural export to another to obtain the best profits on the world market. When world cotton prices rose, they cultivated

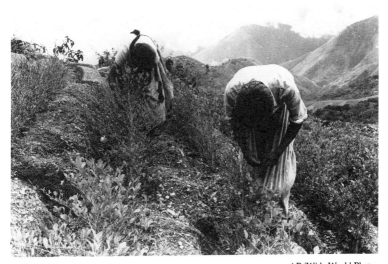

Bolivian farmers tend their hardy coca shrubs on a terraced hillside.

cotton. When cotton prices collapsed in the mid-1970s, they moved into a new growth commodity—cocaine. The shift to the drug trade by Bolivian cotton growers underscores what is now considered a truism: although other Latin American enterprises may fail, drugs always succeed.

Coca must be the world's easiest cash crop to cultivate. It flourishes in poor soil, requires no fertilizer or irrigation, resists blight and pests, produces its first harvest in a year to 18 months and continues to produce for at least 20 years even though its leaves are stripped off four or five times annually. The leaves themselves are nonperishable and lightweight, making transport easy. As for cocaine, the process of transforming coca leaves into the drug is a three-stage process. The first two steps are simple, inexpensive and easily adaptable to almost any work space, from the back of a pickup truck to the inside of an adobe house, and for that reason they are often done by the coca-growing peasants themselves. First, bales of the dried leaves are placed in tubs of water and kerosene and stomped on for several hours. Then the resulting gummy mixture is combined with sulfuric acid, lime, potassium permanganate and more kerosene and squeezed to produce a cream-colored substance known as *pasta básica*, or "basic paste." Pasta básica is the intermediate product from which cocaine is made in the third and final step of the process. The paste is combined with ether and acetone to remove impurities and then filtered to produce a slurry which is dried into a fine white powder—cocaine hydrochloride ($C_{17}H_{21}NO_4HCL$). This final step requires more skill and an investment in chemical solvents not available to peasant processors. It has been done traditionally in a centralized laboratory fed by shipments of pasta básica and controlled by top traffickers, but recently there has been a trend toward hard-to-detect "kitchen sink" labs equipped with microwave ovens.

There are astronomical profits to be made in the cocaine trade, but most of the value is added at the distribution end of the business, as compared to cultivation and refining. The peasants who produce the raw material, coca leaves, typically receive as little as 0.5 percent of the retail price of the final product, cocaine. Even that small percentage is much more than they could earn selling any other crop. Bolivia's *coca-campesinos* soon found themselves with annual incomes as much as 20 times the country's per capita gross national product. But the really big bucks went to the top, creating a cocaine aristocracy that was headed by Santa Cruz cattle rancher Roberto Suárez Gómez, the self-styled King of Cocaine.

Suárez Gómez was an expert pilot who used his fleet of small planes to build an air bridge from the coca fields of Bolivia to cocaine laboratories in Colombia. By 1980 his drug operations were earning him an estimated $400 million a year. A flamboyant figure who carried a gold-plated handgun and kept a pet leopard said to wear a diamond-studded collar, Suárez Gómez fancied himself a modern-day Robin Hood who took from rich Yanqui cocaine consumers to give to poor Bolivians. He funded the education of children in his district while taunting the United States to capture him. Suárez Gómez was only the first top trafficker to polish this folk-hero image.

Colombian Captains of Industry

If Bolivians pioneered the cocaine trade, Colombians turned it into a big business. In a single decade of drug dealing that began in the mid-1970s, the Colombians forged a chaotic criminal activity into a vertically integrated conglomerate that now supplies most of the huge U.S. market. The Colombian traffickers did not force their product on unwilling buyers. U.S. demand attracted Colombian supply. Nevertheless the Colombians, especially the shrewd citizens from the businesswise city of Medellín, brought to trafficking a special organizational talent. They quickly learned how to mass market a product that had been supplied spontaneously. They consolidated lines of supply that reached from coca-growing Bolivia and Peru to their laboratories in Colombia. When foreign coca paste supply could not meet the exploding U.S. demand, they expanded supply by extending coca cultivation in the backlands of Colombia itself. In 1987, 90 percent of the world's coca leaves came from Bolivia and Peru, according to the U.S. government, while 70 to 80 percent of the processed cocaine on the U.S. market came from Colombia, according to Bruce Bagley, an academic expert.

The Colombians revolutionized the way cocaine was smuggled into the United States by replacing human "mules," who "body packed" cocaine across borders, with more-mechanized means of transport that could take full advantage of the growing U.S. market. While serving a marijuana-smuggling sentence in a U.S. prison, Carlos Lehder Rivas dreamed up the scheme of moving cocaine in small private planes and boats. Later the Medellín cocaine cartel of which Lehder was a founding member moved cocaine by the ton in cargo containers carried on freighters. This transport revolution raised the quality and the volume of cocaine in the United States and pushed down its street price so that by 1988 it had fallen to $70–$170 per gram (a gram is 1/28th of an ounce), the lowest point ever.

The lower price of cocaine made it possible and profitable for dealers to develop a new merchandizing item—"crack." Said to be the invention of Jamaican gangs, crack is a boiled-down cocaine residue that can be smoked in small quantities to produce quick

15

euphoria. This cheap and highly addictive form of the drug spread rapidly across the United States. Thus the Colombian traffickers not only took advantage of a business opportunity, they also deepened the U.S. drug problem.

The lure of drug profits many times greater than those that could be made from marijuana set off an explosion of illegal economic activity inside Colombia, eventually generating a powerful, self-conscious group of drug-dealing entrepreneurs. Whatever Colombia gains from the cocaine trade in economic benefits, the country loses in the damage done to its political and social stability by this violent new stratum of cocaine capitalists.

Cocaine and Politics

The South American cocaine trade is centered in three countries, where it involves an estimated one million people, half of them Colombians. These range from peasant coca cultivators to buyers of half-processed coca paste to money-laundering accountants to the top traffickers who employ them. In various statements and documents, the Colombian traffickers have argued that they serve society by creating jobs and generating wealth, but most of the wealth flows toward the top. Unlike the labor-intensive marijuana trade, cocaine trafficking requires substantial capital and tends to concentrate wealth in the hands of a few. The number of those on top is difficult to assess, but one Colombian narcotics expert estimates there are at least 1,000 traffickers with assets worth from $15 million to $200 million. *Forbes* magazine says Pablo Escobar Gaviria, Jorge Luis Ochoa Vásquez and Gonzalo Rodríguez Gacha—the big three of Medellín—have more than $1 billion each. Less is known about Gilberto Rodríguez Orejuela and José Santacruz Londoño, the leaders of the Cali cartel. (The use of the term cartel to describe cocaine-trafficking groups is misleading, since none of them controls the market price.)

These men bring back between $1 billion and $3 billion annually to consume and invest in Colombia. Given the steady devaluation of the Colombian peso, dollar repatriation on this scale is an unsound business practice, but the traffickers are moved by more than the profit motive. They want big bank accounts in Switzerland, but they also want prestige and power back home. They want to launder not only their money but their names. Their lust for legitimacy explains why the Colombian traffickers have invested heavily in politics.

For a while it appeared the emerging cocaine capitalists would buy their way into the inner circles of the country's two major political parties. Both parties accepted drug dollars as campaign donations, and Pablo Escobar, who built up his popularity by playing Robin Hood to Medellín's poor, won a seat in Congress in 1982. He was hounded out by a crusading young senator from the reform wing of the Liberals, Rodrigo Lara Bonilla. Lara Bonilla was murdered in 1984. According to government prosecutors, his two assassins were paid by Pablo Escobar. Lara Bonilla's murder forced Colombia's political elites to confront the traffickers instead of accommodating them, and Colombia's last two presidents have taken strong stands against them.

Although the front door to Colombian party politics is now closed to the traffickers, they may be gaining political power through a side entrance. Farmers' and cattlemen's associations have a lot of political clout in Colombia, and the traffickers have been buying up rural real estate in large amounts, which gives them access to these organizations. It also positions the traffickers to take control of municipal governments, now that a recent political reform has done away with the appointment of Colombia's mayors by the central government in Bogotá and established the local election of these officials.

'Narco-cattlemen'

Drug traffickers have snapped up some 2.5 million acres of farmland, according to one study. The phenomenon is so widespread that the army's main drug fighter, Gen. Jaime Ruiz Barrera, has coined a term for the new landed gentry—narco-cattlemen. In the countryside, their ranches can be identified by the impeccably maintained fences and the ostentatious entryways. The most famous of these belongs to Pablo Escobar, whose Hacienda Nápoles is entered under an arch that holds an actual small plane said to have carried his first cocaine shipment to the United States.

There are many reasons why the narcos are setting themselves up in the countryside. Real estate is an uncomplicated business to enter for the rising new rich unskilled in industrial investments and without access to Colombia's clannish commercial class. Another obvious attraction is security. The rolling hills of a cattle ranch offer good escape routes. Although General Ruiz has a reputation as a tenacious enemy of drug traffickers, he has captured none of them since he was sent to Medellín in early 1988. On one raid the Army found an underground bunker and tunnel system, but the traffickers had fled. Remote ranches can hide not only traffickers but drug laboratories and the clandestine airstrips used to fly out the finished product. In June 1988 General Ruiz's raiders discovered four labs, 2,600 kilograms (5,720 pounds) of cocaine and three airstrips on one of Escobar's ranches on the west bank of the Magdalena River, not far from Hacienda Nápoles.

The middle section of the long Magdalena River Valley that divides Colombia has become a flourishing center for agricultural investments by the traffickers. There the traffickers' rural presence has taken on violent political overtones. Rodríguez Gacha and Fidel Castaño, two fanatically anti-Communist cocaine kings, have built up large cattle ranches in the area. Colombian prosecutors say Castaño and Rodríguez Gacha are using their ranches as training camps for paramilitary groups which the traffickers deploy against villagers who sympathize with leftist guerrillas and the political party they founded, the Patriotic Union. Patriotic Union chairman Jaime Pardo Leal was murdered in October 1987, and the government says his killers were working for Rodríguez Gacha. Pardo's murder was apparently a retaliatory blow for pressure by the guerrillas, who force the traffickers to keep up the price paid peasants for coca paste in the regions under guerrilla control.

The complexity of Colombia's narcopolitics should not obscure the fact that the foundation of the cocaine empire rests on U.S. demand for the drug. As the drug fad of the 1960s became a permanent feature of U.S. life, the steady flow of large amounts of money into the Latin American underground gave rise to a sophisticated, diversified industry—and a new interdependence between Latin America and the United States.

2

Washington's War

Although the United States spends most of its money for drug-law enforcement on domestic police action, the overall antidrug strategy is aimed abroad. This strategy has three components: interdiction—the disruption of drug pipelines; eradication—the destruction of the crops that produce illegal drugs; and extradition—the capture overseas and prosecution in the United States of top drug traffickers, especially Colombians. These remedies are aimed at eliminating or disrupting foreign sources of supply. Drug fighters believe they can "get more bang for the buck" by "going to the source."

During his 1968 presidential campaign Richard M. Nixon promised to do something about crime and permissiveness in U.S. society. Once in the White House, Nixon authorized the first major U.S. attack on Latin American drugs—Operation Intercept. The government's strategy was to pressure Mexico to crack down on marijuana cultivation and trafficking. The tactic was to squeeze the flow of trade and tourists across the U.S.-Mexican border and thus constrict a vital source of Mexican dollar-earnings. U. S. Customs Service agents normally made a cursory inspection of border traffic, but in September 1969 they began subjecting each and every vehicle to a detailed review. Operation Intercept was an economic disaster for Mexico. Mexican farm exports to the United States rotted in the sun as border traffic backed up for miles. U.S. tourist dollars dropped by 70 percent. The Mexican government was outraged, and so were merchants on the U.S. side, since Mexicans stopped coming across to shop. When the Mexican government paved the way for a U.S. retreat by agreeing in principle to crack down on the marijuana trade, Washington called off Operation Intercept after less than a month. Mexican traffickers who had been lying low went back into business.

Victory in Turkey

Nixon had more success when he started fighting the drug war far from U.S. shores. During the 1960s the U.S. use of heroin increased along with the use of all illegal drugs. An estimated 80 percent of the U.S. heroin supply was coming from Turkey, where farmers cultivated opium poppies, the plant from which heroin is derived. Just before Nixon took office, Turkey had agreed to phase out the illegal portion of its opium poppy production, but the Turkish government did not enforce the agreement. Nixon made an issue of it, threatening to cut off U.S. military and economic assistance. As a result, Turkey banned poppy cultivation entirely for two years and then introduced stringent controls to prevent diversion. The Turkish crackdown and the arrest in 1972 of members of a major heroin trafficking ring based in Marseilles, the famous "French connection," blocked the heroin supply line to the United States. (Today Turkey is a major transit route for heroin.)

After the the Nixon Administration closed the door to the East, heroin started coming in from the South, across the Mexican border. By 1973 Mexican peasants had discovered they could increase their income as much as tenfold by cultivating opium poppies. Two years later Mexico was supplying 87 percent of the heroin used in the United States. In late 1975 Mexico started spraying its illegal poppy fields with herbicides, and heroin production shifted to Asia. The new sources of supply were the Golden Crescent countries of Afghanistan, Pakistan and Iran and the Golden Triangle—western Laos, eastern Burma and northern Thailand. The shift in the heroin supply line demonstrates what drug researchers call "the balloon syndrome": when police squeeze drug trafficking in one part of the globe, it pops out in another place and new supply lines are created. This pattern has recurred so many times and in so many parts of the world over the last 15 years that it should be considered an iron law of drug economics. As long as the demand for illegal drugs exists, the huge profits of trafficking will always attract suppliers.

President Nixon had beat the drum against a heroin "epidemic." There is evidence of a substantial increase in U.S. heroin use around 1970, but researchers have questioned whether the use was as widespread as Nixon claimed. They accused his Administration of systematically distorting addiction statistics to create the illusion that Nixon was getting tough with crime in order to strengthen his reelection bid. Governments frequently distort the data on drugs for political reasons. A more serious problem with the Nixon Administration's policy was that the victory of a "get-tough" policy with Turkey was a deceptive success. Turkey was a special case that had little in common with the emerging drug problem in Latin America. First, Turkey produced heroin, and the number of heroin users in the United States was only a fraction of the number of U.S. citizens who would come to use cocaine from Latin America. (There are about 500,000 heroin addicts today, less than one tenth the number of cocaine users.) Second, opium poppies are much easier to eradicate than the hardy coca bush. Third, at the time when the United States threatened to cut off aid to Turkey, that country was embroiled in a bitter dispute with Greece over control of the island of Cyprus. (Turkey invaded Cyprus in 1974.) The potential loss of U.S. military aid outweighed whatever economic benefits were accruing to Turkey from drug dollars. Compliance with the U.S. demand was seen as a matter of national necessity. The situation in Latin America is quite different. Heroin generated fewer

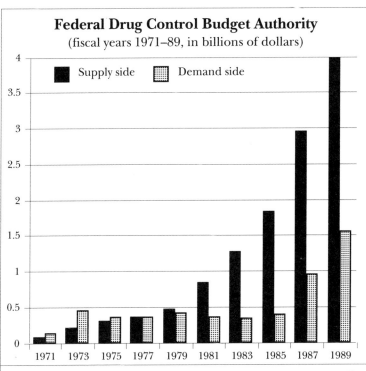

Federal Drug Control Budget Authority
(fiscal years 1971–89, in billions of dollars)

■ Supply side   ▦ Demand side

Supply side: law enforcement, interdiction, investigation, eradication in other countries, international efforts
Demand side: treatment, rehabilitation, education, research

Sources: General Accounting Office and National Drug Policy Board.

profits and had a much smaller impact on the Turkish economy than cocaine would have on the economies of Bolivia, Colombia and Peru. Bolivia and Peru are dependent on cocaine exports to earn the foreign exchange they need to buy their imports.

Sealing South Florida

At his first press conference in March 1981, newly elected President Ronald Reagan said his Administration would refocus U.S. antidrug policy on the demand side of the trafficking equation. "It's far more effective if you take the customers away than if you try to take the drugs away from those who want to be customers," he said. That is probably true, but Reagan never put his words into practice. In fact, his government did quite the opposite from what the President had promised. The Reagan Administration dedicated an unprecedented amount of human and financial resources to repressing drug supply while cutting the funds aimed at reducing drug demand. Federal antidrug spending on law enforcement, interdiction, investigation, eradication and international cooperation had averaged $437 million annually for the preceding five years, but from 1981 to 1986 spending on these supply-side programs more than tripled to an annual average of $1.4 billion. In the same period, funding for the demand-side programs of drug treatment, rehabilitation, education and research fell from an average of $386 million a year to $362.8 million. After the cocaine-related deaths of two prominent athletes stirred a national outcry, Congress intervened in 1986 to increase Federal spending on demand-side programs, but they still received a smaller percentage of total Federal funds than before the Reagan years. Instead of shifting government policy toward the origin of the problem, the demand for drugs, the Reagan Administration remained committed to a law-and-order approach aimed at cutting off supply.

The vanguard of the Reagan attack was the South Florida Task Force, a grandiose interdiction effort that dwarfed anything ever tried before. In January 1982 the Administration reassigned several hundred DEA, Federal Bureau of Investigation, Internal Revenue Service, Customs Service, Bureau of Alcohol, Tobacco and Firearms agents, Treasury Department analysts, Coast Guard personnel and U.S. marshals to antidrug duty in Miami. The city's role as the main U.S. port for Latin American drugs had become obvious when bloody shootouts between trafficking groups had erupted in a Miami shopping center in 1979. Vice President Bush, who was given authority for the Task Force, promised that it would save Miami from "a sea of murders, violence, fear and blood-drenched narcodollars." His chief of operations in this effort was retired Admiral Dan Murphy, who had commanded the U.S. Sixth Fleet. Once in Miami, Murphy proceeded to set up an antidrug armada off southern Florida.

Like all drug statistics, the data on seizures by the Task Force are highly variable. Bush announced in January 1984 that the National Narcotics Border Interdiction System, of which the South Florida Task Force was the centerpiece, had seized almost 5 million pounds of marijuana and 28,000 pounds of cocaine. DEA Administrator Francis Mullen, who resented the Task Force as an intrusion of politicians into law enforcement, said it could claim credit for the seizure of only 2 million pounds of marijuana and 8,000 pounds of cocaine. Whatever the numbers, there is little reason to doubt that the Task Force was capturing large amounts of drugs, but this did not mean that it had cordoned off Miami. Cocaine was pouring into the city. In fact, there was so much cocaine that it glutted the Miami market. Wholesale prices dropped from $60,000 per kilo in 1982, when the Task Force was established, to under $13,000–$20,000 in 1989. What had happened? Why did cocaine prices collapse at a time when U.S. demand was growing?

Traffickers Switch to Cocaine

Many experts believe that the answer can be found in government policy itself. They say that by attempting to seal the border, the Reagan Administration unwittingly prodded traffickers to switch from smuggling Colombian marijuana to smuggling cocaine, thus increasing supply and lowering prices. As James Lieber pointed out in *The Atlantic* in 1986, the legal risks for both drugs were equal. Florida imposed the same mandatory prison sentences for trafficking in either marijuana or cocaine. And if detection was the measure, the risk of getting caught was less with cocaine than with marijuana. A kilo of cocaine with the same market value as a ton of marijuana could be concealed in the bottom of a suitcase whereas the marijuana required a boat or a plane to move it around, making it a bigger target for the Task Force.

While it cannot be said for certain that this is the correct explanation for the spurt in the supply of cocaine, there is little

25

doubt that the Administration's stepped-up interdiction of marijuana, especially that portion arriving in boats and planes from Colombia, stimulated U.S. citizens to grow their own. The demand for domestic marijuana had been kept down by its high cost— three or four times that of the imported variety. After the Task Force launched its attack on foreign supply, "homegrown" became a billion-dollar agribusiness that now supplies a quarter of the U.S. marijuana market. The National Organization for the Reform of Marijuana Laws concludes from this that "the South Florida Task Force helped create the market conditions which spurred domestic production." One former Colombian president has archly observed that the expansion of the U.S. marijuana supply is a classic example of import substitution: the U.S. barred Colombian competition and thus boosted its own fledgling industry.

Extraditing Colombian Traffickers

If interdiction was the key weapon in the Reagan Administration's antidrug arsenal at home, extradition was the big gun abroad. In 1979 the Carter Administration negotiated with Colombia an agreement to extradite its citizens to the United States for prosecution for 33 crimes, ranging from tax evasion to drug trafficking. The agreement deviated from prevailing international law by allowing deportation from the country of citizenship. It also overrode an existing Colombian law that expressly prohibited such a practice. But President Julio César Turbay Ayala was willing to take exceptional measures against drug traffickers. In his inaugural address in 1978 Turbay had declared war on drugs. Three months later he had sent the military into the Guajira Peninsula, which was riddled with clandestine airstrips serving the Florida marijuana market. Turbay left office before an extradition case came across his desk, however, and it fell to his successor, Belisario Betancur Cuartas, to deal with what would become a subject of heated debate and a motive for murder.

Colombian popular opinion did not share Turbay's enthusiasm for extradition. The treaty had been drawn up with marijuana traffickers in mind, but most Colombians believed that fighting marijuana not only damaged the country's economic interests but corrupted the drug fighters as well. The National Police was receiving an estimated $110 million annually in marijuana protection money, according to Bagley. The military ordered Army troops out of the Guajira before the same thing happened to them. In the United States police had eased up on marijuana arrests. President Jimmy Carter had urged Congress to abolish criminal penalties for possessing an ounce of the drug. With such a lenient attitude in the White House, why should Colombia get tough with traffickers?

Betancur took office in 1982, after Reagan had replaced Carter in the White House. A few months later Colombian police, acting on a request from the U.S. embassy, arrested two men accused of smuggling marijuana to Miami. Reagan's ambassador, Lewis Tambs, pushed for their extradition, but Betancur was a moderate nationalist who favored an independent foreign policy, and he objected to the extradition treaty as an incursion into his country's sovereignty. Betancur let the extradition orders remain unsigned.

While the president delayed his decision, cocaine traffickers began to demonstrate their emerging political power by stirring up popular opinion against the treaty. The traffickers took out newspaper ads and sponsored a series of public forums at which politicians and legal authorities, including a former Supreme Court justice, inveighed against extradition as an imposition of the gringos. Some of the speakers at these forums wanted to ingratiate themselves with the narco new rich, but others were honestly concerned about the issue of U.S. interference in Colombian legal affairs. Colombia has a strong legal tradition backed by a constitution that is 103 years old. Colombians are not particularly anti-American, but they have had a distrust of U.S. foreign policy ever since President Theodore Roosevelt engineered the secession of the Colombian department of Panama. Opposition to the extradition treaty spread to the streets. The slogan "Colombia, Don't Hand Over Your Sons" circulated widely.

Although Betancur was uncooperative on extradition, he was

not indifferent to the problem of drug trafficking. He appointed as his justice minister Lara Bonilla, who had personally hounded out of Parliament Pablo Escobar. As a minister, Lara Bonilla continued his antidrug crusade by grounding 300 planes that flew drugs to the United States and by proposing a regional pact to halt drug trafficking. His efforts stirred the ire of the traffickers, and in February 1984 one of his assistants, an outspoken advocate of the U.S.-Colombian extradition treaty, was killed by assassins. Lara Bonilla himself received death threats, and Ambassador Tambs gave him a bulletproof jacket. The jacket did not save his life. In April 1984 he was murdered on a Bogotá street by two killers on motorcycles, probably in reprisal for the police raid seven weeks before on the massive cocaine laboratory known as Tranquilandia. The police commander who led the raid was later gunned down.

The murder of his justice minister shocked President Betancur into reconsidering his stand on extradition, and he soon thereafter signed six deportation orders. It was not an easy decision. "As a law professor I taught for more than 30 years that we have the right to be judged by our own laws in our own country," Betancur told an interviewer. "But we are fighting with scarce resources against an international mafia that is threatening the very security of the Colombian state." During the next two years Betancur's government would deport 10 Colombian traffickers to the United States. These extradition orders came at a high price. The judges and government officials who approved extradition requests were routinely murdered.

Law, Order and a Revolving Door

Violence was not the only weapon the traffickers used against extradition. They tried to negotiate a way out. At a meeting in Panama in May 1984 they offered to dismantle their drug empire and pay off Colombia's $11 billion foreign debt if the government revised the treaty. Betancur backed away from the deal after a storm of protest arose when Tambs leaked the offer to the press.

The Reagan Administration was adamant in defense of extradition. The DEA saw the solution to the drug-trafficking problem in law-and-order terms. Prosecution in the United States was the only effective weapon against the traffickers because they could buy or bludgeon their way out of any jail in Colombia. And since Colombians dominated the entire South American cocaine trade, the DEA hoped that their extradition would destabilize the drug empire. But the cocaine trade was much more than a law enforcement issue. Cocaine smuggling had become a vast transnational business that could not be bankrupted by jailing top traffickers and snuffing out crime "families." The Medellín cartel's decentralized hierarchy was stronger than its individual leaders. Arrests simply created new room at the top, and ambitious narcos moved into the jobs of those jailed. In February 1987 Colombian police captured Lehder. In a great victory for the DEA, Lehder was sent to the United States for trial, but his place was promptly filled by Rodríguez Gacha.

The traffickers feared the U.S. justice system, but it was not fear alone that gave rise to their furious reaction to the threat of extradition. Extradition enraged the traffickers because it branded them as criminals and second-class citizens, and not as the successful businessmen they saw themselves to be. After the Lara Bonilla murder, Colombia's traditional elites turned away from the traffickers and lined up behind Betancur on the extradition issue. The traffickers responded by attacking Colombia's elites as unpatriotic "sellouts" to "North American imperialism." The United States pushed the confrontation to the breaking point by making extradition the axis around which pivoted not only U.S. antidrug policy in Colombia but U.S.-Colombian relations. In December 1987 Ochoa Vásquez, a Medellín cocaine magnate, bribed or threatened his way out of a Bogotá jail before the Colombian government could deport him to the United States. The United States retaliated by delaying visas to Colombian travelers and by holding up at the border perishable Colombian exports such as shrimp and flowers. Under pressure from Washington, President Virgilio Barco Vargas promised to pursue Ochoa. Cornered, the traffickers murdered Attorney General Carlos Mauro Hoyos, a strong advocate of extradition. They then kidnapped Bogotá mayoral candidate Andrés Pastrana, the son of

29

a former president and thus a symbol of Colombia's traditional political class. In defense of the kidnapping, the traffickers issued an indignant communiqué that read like a manifesto for the narco new rich. Calling themselves "the Extraditables," they attacked the elites for betraying patriotic Colombians and declared "total war" on the government. Bloodied, and worried about the destabilizing effects of constant attacks on its authority, the Barco government eased up on its extradition efforts.

The matter took a new twist the following October when the U.S. Congress passed an antidrug law that imposed capital punishment on murderous drug traffickers. Colombia does not have capital punishment so it cannot extradite its citizens, traffickers included, on capital charges unless the president invokes state-of-siege powers. In effect, Congress restricted extradition. After years of pushing Colombia to turn over its drug traffickers, the United States itself eroded the policy, but not before many Colombians had died to defend it. In retrospect, the extradition strategy appears to have been a complete failure: The Extraditables are still in business; huge volumes of illegal drugs continue to flow from Colombia to the United States; the reprisals imposed after Ochoa's release scarred U.S.-Colombian relations; and the rule of law is no stronger in Colombia than before. Instead of destabilizing the drug cartels, extradition helped destabilize Colombia.

Decertification

As drug abuse became a U.S. political issue in the mid-1980s, members of Congress started challenging Reagan Administration policy, which seemed unable to smother the explosion of cocaine use. Simmering discontent on Capitol Hill turned into a full-blown revolt after basketball star Len Bias and the Cleveland Browns' defensive back Don Rogers both died of cocaine overdoses in the same month, June 1986. The mass media, which in the past had frequently glamorized cocaine use, began emphasizing its dangers. People across the country demanded action, and congressmen rushed to legislate. The result was a $1.7 billion omnibus drug bill that filled 56 pages of the *Congressional Record* and tried to reach into every phase of illegal drug production and consumption, at home and abroad.

Many sections of the bill touched on aspects of the Latin American drug trade, but one provision injected Congress directly into drug diplomacy. Since 1972, the Rodino amendment had authorized the President to cut off military and economic aid to any country that failed to work to control illegal narcotics. The 1986 bill changed the law to require that 50 percent of the direct foreign aid for some two dozen drug-producing or transit countries be automatically withheld at the start of each fiscal year. It was then up to the President to tell Congress whether or not these countries had "cooperated fully" in the antidrug effort during the previous year. Any country "decertified" by the President not only lost its aid but could be the target of a U.S. veto on loan requests to multinational lending agencies. Congress could override the President's choices and impose its own list of which countries should be rewarded and which should be punished. The result is an annual series of congressional hearings in which U.S. congressmen and State Department officials argue about the shortcomings of foreign governments (but rarely their own). These debates are reported overseas, where commentators pointedly note that the United States casts blame abroad while failing to eradicate its marijuana fields at home.

Under the threat of decertification, Bolivia finally agreed in 1987 to eradicate coca grown for export, but it, unlike such Latin American drug producers as Mexico and Colombia, is a small, powerless country vulnerable to U.S. pressure. In any case, the Bolivian government has had a hard time translating its words into action. Coca cultivation continues to flourish. The threat of decertification is not only ineffective, it is demeaning to the United States' Latin American allies. During the hearings some congressmen cannot resist the opportunity to give their southern neighbors a verbal thrashing. While these speeches may reassure constituents that their congressman is "doing something about drugs," they often demonstrate a faulty knowledge of Latin American reality. During the 1988 decertification debate Representative Larry Smith (D-Fla.), chairman of the House Foreign Affairs

Committee's Task Force on International Narcotics Control, led an attempt to ban aid to one Caribbean and four Latin American drug-producing or transiting countries, including Peru. Smith contended that Peru should be punished because, among other things, it was "a country which has never successfully prosecuted any drug traffickers." In fact, at the moment Smith was delivering his speech on the House floor, a Peruvian cocaine trafficker who had once had extensive influence in the ruling political party was serving a 15-year sentence in Lima's Canto Grande Prison. Another top trafficker was awaiting trial while Peruvian investigators unraveled his connections in the military and the police.

State Department's Criteria

Ultimately Smith was voted down and the State Department's list of which countries should and should not receive aid prevailed. The list demonstrates how U.S. foreign-policy makers have yoked the drug issue to other agendas. The Reagan Administration never asked Congress to decertify a foreign ally, no matter how deeply that country's government might have been embroiled in the drug trade. For example, the regime of former Paraguayan dictator Gen. Alfredo Stroessner was thoroughly enmeshed in drug trafficking and money laundering, but the State Department said Paraguay should be certified on "national interest" grounds. In February 1989 Stroessner was overthrown by Gen. Andrés Rodríquez. Rodríguez was linked to drugs by foreign diplomats, academicians and media reports of a State Department document that accused him of being the country's number one trafficker. Nevertheless, a month after his coup, the State Department once again asked Congress to certify Paraguay. Honduras has been part of the Medellín network for years, and DEA officials believe military officers are involved in the trade. The State Department never demanded sanctions against Honduras, however, probably because it was a vital staging area for the U.S.-backed Nicaraguan contra rebels. There is strong evidence that the contras themselves were involved in trafficking, possibly with the collaboration of U.S. covert agents. The justification for ignoring trafficking by U.S. friends is the East-West conflict. The

United States is willing to look the other way as long as the drug traffickers are anti-Communist. An example of this principle was the shift in Washington's attitude toward Panamanian strongman Gen. Manuel Antonio Noriega. According to the sworn testimony of José Blandón, a former Panamanian intelligence official, the United States had known for years that Noriega was doing drug business, but he was considered a useful asset as an informer for the Central Intelligence Agency (CIA) and a prop for the contras. Blandón told a Senate subcommittee in February 1988 that Noriega was a double agent who had worked not only for the CIA and the contras but for Fidel Castro and the Sandinistas as well. Three weeks after Blandón's testimony, President Reagan asked Congress to decertify Panama, and it did. President Bush made the same request in 1989.

Drugs and National Security

As the 1980s progressed the Reagan Administration merged the war on drugs with the cold war. The first to ideologize openly the antidrug effort was U.S. ambassador to Colombia Tambs. In 1984 Tambs coined the term narcoguerrilla to describe a presumed alliance between narcotraficantes and Communist guerrillas. In fact these two groups more often than not had opposing interests. The guerrillas wanted to overthrow the Colombian system while the traffickers wanted to take a place at the top of it. For a while this conflict in long-term goals was muted by the fact that Colombian coca was grown in territory controlled by the guerrillas. Thus the traffickers were forced to cooperate with the guerrillas and pay them a "war tax" on coca paste. But Colombian coca was of poor quality, and as cultivation expanded in Bolivia and Peru, traffickers turned away from it and abandoned their agreements with the guerrillas. By late 1988 paramilitary groups organized by the traffickers were attacking guerrilla strongholds in Colombia.

In 1986 the Administration had officially identified the drug trade as a national security threat to the United States. Citing "undeniable" links between drug trafficking and terrorism, a presidential directive issued in April of that year authorized the

U.S. military to fight drugs in other countries. Three months later, six Black Hawk helicopters, four small planes and 170 U.S. troops led by Vietnam War hero Gen. John Taylor arrived in Santa Cruz, Bolivia, to accompany DEA agents and Bolivian antidrug police in attacks on cocaine production. In 18 weeks of raids, the campaign, known as Operation Blast Furnace, destroyed 16 labs and seized four tons of coca paste but was able to arrest only one 17-year-old boy because the traffickers were tipped off before every mission. Despite its impressive military technology, Operation Blast Furnace made no lasting impact on the Bolivian cocaine industry. Local prices paid for coca paste dropped briefly while supply lines were disrupted, but prices rose to previous levels once the raiders had returned home to the Southern Command in Panama. They left behind some political fallout. Drug raids in the drug-dependent Chapare and Beni regions had stirred up massive local protests. Leftist labor officials and the leaders of the farmers' federation organized protests in front of the U.S. embassy where peasants chanted "Long live coca!" In Bolivia's Congress, opposition parties accused the government of surrendering national sovereignty to the Yanqui invaders and warned that the United States was using the drug issue as a cover for a permanent military presence in Bolivia. The notion seemed farfetched until a Southern Command document, leaked to the press in 1987, confirmed that the Pentagon sees the Beni region as a possible staging area to fight low-intensity conflicts in South America's heartland. Since then the United States has encouraged Bolivia to build bases there, and U.S. troops have returned for joint maneuvers and civic projects.

Peru: A Case Study

If the Pentagon's real interest in South America is not drugs but counterinsurgency, the immediate focus of that interest is more likely to be Peru than Bolivia. Events in Peru are rapidly escaping the control of the central government in Lima, raising the possibility that the United States will try to fill the power vacuum. And in Peru, as in Bolivia, the path to military intervention is being paved by the U.S. antidrug effort.

In 1980 a Peruvian Maoist group with the ponderous name of "The Communist Party of Peru—for the Shining Path of José Carlos Mariátegui" opted for armed struggle in the southern Andean province of Ayacucho. Since then "Shining Path" has moved out of its mountain redoubt and into the whole country, advancing from 129 armed attacks in 1980 to 2,552 in 1987, according to the Interior Ministry. With a penchant for violence and an estimated 5,000 militants and 20,000 active supporters, Shining Path has virtually pushed Peru to the edge of a total civil war.

In late 1983 Shining Path sent cadres into the upper end of the Huallaga River Valley, 225 miles northeast of Lima. Locals call the valley the "eyebrow of the jungle" because it is a green edge of the Amazon Basin pushed up against the stark slopes of the Andes, but the valley is known to the world as the cradle of the cocaine trade. Coca cultivation arrived with the first settlers in the 1930s. They sold their legal crops to a state monopoly, and by 1960 there were 3,000 members of the valley coca producers' association. Ten years later farmers started moving into coca cultivation in large numbers. The cause was the voracious American demand for cocaine. In 1978 U.S. cocaine consumption had climbed to between 19 and 25 tons, according to a U.S. government interagency group. By 1984 it had grown to between 71 and 137 tons. That would be an increase of more than 700 percent in six years. Today between one third and one half of the world's coca leaf is grown in the 540-square-mile Upper Huallaga, making it the world's primary producer.

Press accounts published in Peru and in the United States suggest that Shining Path went to the Upper Huallaga in pursuit of drug profits. Interviews with travelers in the guerrilla-controlled countryside confirm that Shining Path "taxes" coca farmers. These sources say the guerrillas use the funds to pay for medicines and civic projects needed by the villagers themselves. There is a persistent rumor that the guerrillas are charging the traffickers "landing fees" to use clandestine airstrips, but there is no evidence that the organization is getting rich on coca dollars. In fact Shining Path is fanatically committed to a Maoist ideology that makes a virtue out of staying poor and fighting a "people's war" with dynamite stolen from the mines and weapons taken from the security forces. Gustavo Gorriti, the Peruvian journalist who has written a book on Shining Path, says it is probably the poorest group of guerrillas in the world.

It is more likely that the guerrillas went to the Upper Huallaga not to fatten their war chests but to make war on the enemy—the U.S. antidrug campaign. Analysts say the rebels have dealt themselves in as key players in the valley by defending the coca-growing campesinos from government antidrug operations while mediating disputes between the growers and their Colombian buyers. Coca cultivation is the basis of the valley economy. Some 20,000 to 60,000 families are involved. Attempts to eradicate coca and eliminate the drug trade from the valley throw farmers into "a panic," according to the director of the U.S.-financed coca eradication project based in Tingo María. Shining Path exploits these fears. "Death to the DEA" is one of the slogans seen most often in guerrilla-controlled parts of the valley.

Aided by the cooperation of the Peruvian government, particularly under President Alan García, the United States has been more directly involved in fighting drugs in the Upper Huallaga than anywhere else in South America, and the presence of Shining Path guerrillas in the valley complicates the U.S. effort. The large U.S. antidrug program walks on two legs: agricultural development and law enforcement.

The U.S. Agency for International Development (AID) tries to persuade Upper Huallaga Valley peasants to grow something besides coca. To this end AID has spent $20 million since 1983 and has another $4.5 million budgeted for the next three years. (Peru has put another $11 million into the project.) With this money the agency has provided agricultural extension services to some 1,200 valley farmers who, it says, have given up cultivating coca and now produce coffee, cacao, bananas and other crops. This is only a tiny fraction of the rising number of coca-cultivating peasants, and there are doubts that even the farmers in the AID program have kicked the coca habit. Peruvian AID workers told a *Washington Post* correspondent in 1984 that some

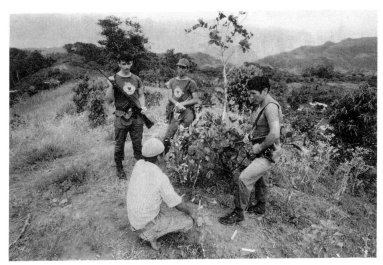

**Shining Path guerrillas in Tingo María, Peru,
look on as coca shrubs are dug up at government orders.**

of the farmers they were helping with their rice crops still continued to grow coca in nearby fields.

As for antidrug police action, over the last decade the State Department's Narcotics Assistance Unit in the Lima embassy has injected $31 million into Peruvian drug enforcement, mostly in the Upper Huallaga Valley. This money has paid the salaries of two sets of people: the squad of 460 manual laborers hired to eradicate coca plots by hand; and the Peruvian antidrug police, who number about 500. In 1987 the eradication program had ground to a halt and Shining Path guerrillas had reemerged as a potent force in the Upper Huallaga Valley. The Peruvian Army had controlled the valley under a government-declared state of emergency from July 1984 to December 1985. It had rolled back Shining Path but allowed drug trafficking to flourish. Interior Ministry officials say Army officers had taken large payoffs from traffickers. With the encouragement of the U.S. embassy in Lima, the government decided in 1987 to put the southern half of the valley under control of the police. According to farmers, travelers, Peruvian government officials, church workers and United Nations community workers interviewed by the author during a five-day trip through the Upper Huallaga Valley in May 1988, Shining Path dominated dozens of tiny villages and strongly influenced several large towns. Police could no longer patrol the roads. Traffic was halted frequently by Shining Path cadres who lectured drivers and painted their vehicles with the hammer-and-sickle symbol.

Because the Peruvian police are funded by the U.S. government, advised by DEA strategists and transported by U.S.-provided Bell helicopters flown by U.S. and Peruvian pilots, the United States is in danger of being drawn into a full-blown counterinsurgency war. Craig Chretien, the DEA country attaché for Peru, says "it's difficult, but not impossible" to sort out traffickers from guerrillas, but he says his officers have never been involved in any firefights with Shining Path. (DEA agents are legally prohibited from antiguerrilla actions.) Gorriti believes Shining Path may be trying to precipitate U.S. military intervention in order to mobilize Peru against the Yanquis.

Controversial Spike

One way the United States has tried to avoid an open confrontation is by taking to the air. The antidrug police now travel only in helicopters. Dropping herbicides from planes instead of pulling up coca plants by hand would be the logical next step. The United States carries out herbicide attacks on marijuana and opium in seven countries, but it has had trouble finding a chemical that kills the indomitable coca shrub. In October 1987 Agriculture Department experts tried a new tack. Working on test plots in the Upper Huallaga, they applied herbicides to the roots of coca plants and came up with two killers. One of them, tibuthiuron, which is marketed by Eli Lilly & Co. under the trademark Spike, was quietly selected by the State Department to bombard valley coca plantations. Peruvian President García appeared ready to approve the State Department plan. (García is a fiercer foe of drug trafficking than one would expect, given Peru's dependence on drug dollars.) Then U.S. environmental experts, including a longtime Agriculture Department official who resigned in protest, said Spike posed serious health and ecology hazards, and Lilly refused to cooperate with the State Department. The herbicide issue, which had been kept under wraps by both Washington and Lima, exploded in the Peruvian press in June 1988. Now García insists that Spike must be approved by UN experts before it can be dropped on the Upper Huallaga. The State Department says Spike is safe but that it is also considering other herbicides. Peru's interior minister says Spike should be used but that the United States will have to provide $600 million to relocate coca-growing peasants in other occupations.

Whether or not a coca-killing herbicide is ultimately dropped on the Upper Huallaga, Shining Path is actively using the issue as an organizing tool. In August 1988 Shining Path staged a three-day "armed strike" against the use of Spike, which it denounced by name in leaflets circulated in the region. The strike completely paralyzed commerce in the towns in the valley and shut down traffic on its main highway. An unconfirmed newspaper report said 10 people died in confrontations with authorities. A U.S. helicopter pilot was hit by small-arms fire.

Any analysis of the cost-effectiveness of the U.S. campaign in the Upper Huallaga Valley would have to find it a failure. Despite the best efforts of the United States, coca cultivation, formerly concentrated around the town of Tingo María, has spread all over the valley. In 10 years the area involved has increased sixfold, to 280,000 acres, according to State Department figures. The Peruvian antidrug police say the actual amount is almost twice that. Of course the $50 million the United States has spent to fight cocaine trafficking in the Upper Huallaga is a tiny amount in comparison with the estimated $15 billion U.S. citizens snorted and smoked away on cocaine consumption in 1988. The issue is not the amount of money, but the tendency for it to increase. As Upper Huallaga coca cultivation expands, Washington throws more and more tax dollars at an intractable problem. Drug-enforcement aid to Peru has more than quadrupled since 1985, and Washington has even bigger plans for the future. The United States is now carving out a base camp deep in the heart of cocaine country and intends to station American personnel there.

The U.S. antidrug campaign in Peru's Upper Huallaga Valley offers an example of the dangers of trying to "micromanage" the complex political economy of a coca-growing region. In attempting to isolate and eliminate coca cultivation with a carrot-and-stick policy, the United States has softened up the valley's resistance to Shining Path. Residents are not enamored of the guerrillas, whose systematic use of terror permits no opposition. But faced with a choice between guerrilla terror and the loss of their livelihoods, farmers are apt to choose survival. Any U.S. attempt to set up a massive economic adjustment program that would wean the valley from its coca dependence would be not only costly but risky, since Shining Path would target the program for attack. Only time will tell if Washington can resist the logic of an antidrug policy that seems destined to pull the United States deeper into Peru's guerrilla war. Like all wars, the war on drugs will be harder to end than it was to begin.

3

A Joint Venture

For many years the inter-American debate about drugs was a dialogue of the deaf. Each side moralistically accused the other of causing the problem while trying to minimize its own responsibilities. This exercise in hurling blame became pointless as the line blurred between drug-consuming and drug-producing nations. Both sides have become enmeshed in all aspects of the trade. North Americans produce tons of marijuana. Latin Americans consume large amounts of cocaine products. Both derive financial benefits from the drug trade. Both are damaged by its corrosive effects. Drug trafficking has become a joint venture that spans and unites the hemisphere.

Latin Americans read with great interest news stories about the U.S. marijuana industry. Wire-service reports that marijuana farming is a billion-dollar agribusiness in the United States get good play in Latin American newspapers and frequently end up on editorial pages. The thrust of editorial comment, especially in the marijuana-growing nations of Colombia and Mexico, is that Uncle Sam is a hypocrite. Washington pressures Latin American nations to spray marijuana with herbicides that are not used in the United States. The United States expects Latin America to eliminate drugs root and branch while authorities in Arkansas and California cannot even cut down the marijuana plants flourishing in roadside ditches. Where they have been successful, growers have simply moved indoors. If Congress were to apply to state governments the same standards it uses to judge foreign governments in the annual decertification hearings, more than one governor would find his Federal funds in jeopardy.

U.S. Policy Suspect

Observing the U.S. double standard on marijuana, the most cynical Latin American analysts conclude that Washington conducts a calculated policy of eliminating competition from foreign marijuana suppliers to protect domestic producers. A more widespread opinion is that it is politically easier for Washington to fight drugs overseas than at home, where there are 20 million marijuana consumers. If the colossus of the North cannot defeat its homegrown traffickers, how can the much-weaker Latin American governments stand up to the guns of the mighty Medellín cartel?

This logic undermines Latin America's will to fight drugs. Thus U.S. embassies in Latin America have stressed Washington's efforts to eradicate marijuana while downplaying the extent of U.S. cultivation. The State Department has placed special emphasis on defeating the claim that "marijuana is America's largest cash crop," attributing it to statistics deliberately inflated by the marijuana legalization lobby. To this end the United States Information Service (USIS) distributed in early 1988 a press release listing the five most important harvests of the year before, measured by dollar value. Marijuana was not one of them. In its release the USIS quoted an Agriculture Department spokesman who said that the cash value of marijuana could not be calculated "since it's difficult to measure an illegal crop." This circular reasoning, that marijuana was not a top U.S. cash crop because its value could not be calculated, did not stand the test of time.

In a March 30, 1988, memo to all Federal prosecutors, Attorney General Edwin Meese 3d instructed them to adopt a "more consistent enforcement presence on the demand side." During his April visit to South America, Meese was told by many leaders that the United States was soft on drugs. In May President Reagan launched the zero-tolerance program, and the State Department followed suit. The department's new line not only stressed Washington's determination to eliminate home-grown marijuana but acknowledged that the problem was enormous in scope. (The DEA expects the United States to be the world's largest producer by the early 1990s and to begin exporting soon thereafter.) The State Department implemented its more open policy by organizing a tour of U.S. marijuana sites for Colombian journalists. After his return one of them wrote a report headlined "Drugs Made in USA."

Latin American Drug Use Soars

If Washington has moved away from its sanctimonious stance on drug production, Latin America has come to admit that drug consumption is not a problem for the Yanquis alone. At one time top Colombian trafficker Lehder could boast that cocaine would be Latin America's "atomic bomb" against North American society, but cocaine use has now exploded in all three of the South American source countries and spread to the transshipping nations of Venezuela, Paraguay, Argentina and the Caribbean.

The most common mode of consumption is cigarettes laced with pasta básica, the intermediary product between coca and cocaine. Called basuco in Colombia, pastillo in Peru and simply pitillo (cigarette) in Bolivia, pasta básica cigarettes are a poor man's version of the crack cocaine used in the United States. Like crack, pasta básica is cheap and produces an intense, short-lived "high" that leaves the user hungry for more. But unlike the cocaine from which crack is made, pasta básica is not refined. It contains lethal impurities such as lead, sulphuric acid and kerosene, and experts consider it to be much more harmful to human health than crack.

Basuco consumption emerged in Colombia in two stages. First, traffickers encouraged the cultivation of the low-grade Colombian variety of coca to meet escalating U.S. demand. Second, when higher-quality foreign coca came on line, the traffickers dumped the domestic crop inside Colombia in the form of basuco. In 1987 Colombia's Health Ministry estimated that 300,000 to 500,000 of the country's 28 million residents smoked basuco regularly. A UN report says its use in Colombia is one of the world's worst drug problems, and Colombian leaders now frankly acknowledge that their country has a serious habit.

In Bolivia the consumption of coca is no longer limited to the benign practice of chewing its leaves. An estimated 20 percent of Bolivian youth between the ages of 14 and 24 have a pitillo problem. Santa Cruz, Bolivia's second-largest city, has dozens of "smoking houses" patronized by teenagers and young professionals. In Cochabamba, gateway to the Chapare coca-growing region, there are as many as 800 to 1,000 young children who smoke pitillo. A drug rehabilitation center director in Cochabamba traces the problem back to the U.S. drug interdiction effort Operation Blast Furnace. When traffickers could not export pasta básica, they used it to pay workers and sold it to local consumers. This explanation provides an insight into the unexpected side effects of interdiction, but it does not tell why Bolivians all across the country are consuming as much as 100 tons of pasta básica annually.

Bolivian leaders are not always eager to discuss drug consumption. One official told a UN drug hearing in February 1988 that reports of expanding drug use in Bolivia were unjustified and could hurt the country's image as a drug-fighting nation. Perhaps he was referring to Bolivia's image in the decertification hearings to be held in the U.S. Congress the following month. If so, his fears were justified. During the hearings a subcommittee chairman urged Congress to withhold foreign aid to Bolivia because it had not done enough about drugs. Such threats may produce formal compliance but they will not generate a will to fight drugs.

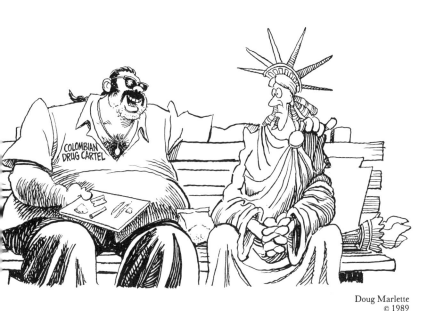

Doug Marlette
© 1989
New York Newsday

"Your lips say 'no, no,' but your nose says 'yes, yes'!"

A better way would be to quietly and convincingly call the attention of Bolivia's leaders to the undeniable evidence that pitillo smoking is becoming epidemic.

A good model for U.S. drug diplomacy in Bolivia would be the U.S.-funded drug prevention program in Peru. The Center of Information and Education for the Prevention of Drug Abuse, or CEDRO, not only reaches into barrio communities but conducts informational seminars for Peruvian political figures. In both of these efforts CEDRO wisely maintains a low-profile approach that avoids direct confrontations on policy questions while raising awareness of the implications of increasing pasta básica consumption.

Wherever it may occur, large-scale drug trafficking and abuse create significant public health, criminal justice and social problems. In the United States the scars are obvious in such places as

New York City's midtown bus terminal, where 200,000 passengers a day must pass through a maze of crack, crime and homelessness. Behind the jarring images are a mind-numbing series of statistics: cocaine-related hospital emergencies in the United States increased fivefold from 1982 to 1986; cocaine wars caused homicides to jump 70 percent in 1988 in Washington, D.C., making it the murder capital of the country; one third of the 44,000 Federal prisoners are serving time for drug-related offenses; more than half of New York City's heroin addicts are infected with the fatal AIDS virus; every year 375,000 infants are exposed to health-threatening drugs. Reliable social statistics are harder to come by in Latin America, but it is likely that the same grim trends can be found south of the border.

Mutual Impact

Drug dollars generate corruption and violence in both the United States and Latin America. The power of drug dollars has made the U.S. criminal justice system more corrupt than at any other time since Prohibition, according to law enforcement specialists. Sheriffs in several Georgia counties have been implicated in trafficking. (Traffickers started landing their planes in Georgia after the crackdown by the South Florida Task Force.) Dozens of police officers in Miami and New York City have come under investigation. At the Federal level, 20 U.S. Customs Service agents were charged after a corruption probe in 1986. Two more were arrested in December 1988 and accused of belonging to a Colombian drug ring. Three former DEA officials have been charged with conspiring to deal cocaine and launder drug profits. *The New York Times* reported that even a veteran FBI agent has confessed to selling cocaine. Many believe that these and other corruption cases now in the courts are only the tip of the iceberg.

As for violence, almost all of the U.S. fatalities result from shoot-outs between rival traffickers, but their escalating firepower turns poor neighborhoods into free-fire zones. Occasionally a policeman dies. The drug-related murder of New York City

Patrolman Edward Byrne in March 1988 provoked a national outrage. Other fronts in the shooting war on drugs are U.S. national forests, where rangers were assaulted by marijuana growers 75 times in 1987. These and other data about drugs were bandied about during the 1988 U.S. presidential campaign, stirring widespread outrage against the traffickers. *Newsweek* called it the perception that "they've got Uzis [submachine guns], and they're everywhere."

There is cause for concern, but no one believes that traffickers are taking over in the United States. Latin America, however, has already had one "cocaine coup" and others may be on the way. Financed by the cocaine clans, Bolivian Gen. Luis García Meza staged a coup in July 1980 and put the Interior Ministry under the control of the cousin of Roberto Suárez Gómez, the "King of Cocaine." For the next year García Meza's outlaw regime raked in revenues earned by taxing cocaine shipments while giving free rein to Nazi war criminals like Klaus Barbie, who was entertained in the presidential palace as an official guest. García Meza was eventually overthrown by officers unhappy that he had made Bolivia a pariah in the world. A more enduring mix of drugs and military men can be found in Panama, where General Noriega has managed to rule from behind the scenes since 1983 despite charges of drug trafficking, money laundering and racketeering.

Both Sides Suffer . . .

These two flamboyant cases should not obscure the constant, grinding erosion of Latin American political systems by drug trafficking. Drug-related violence and corruption bore into Latin America's fragile democracies, posing a threat not only to the stability of these countries but to the national security of the United States as well. It is the damage done to Latin American democratic institutions, rather than any supposed narcoguerrilla alliance, that makes drug trafficking a national security danger to the United States.

The institution of democracy rests on the rule of laws, not men, but the ruthless and wealthy traffickers mock legal authority and impose personal systems of "justice" administered by paid killers. One dramatic example was the assassination attempt against former Colombian Justice Minister Enrique Parejo González. After signing 10 extradition orders against traffickers, Parejo tried to escape reprisals by taking a diplomatic post in Hungary, but in January 1987 he was shot near his home in Budapest. Parejo miraculously recovered, but the Colombian legal system remains seriously injured by this and hundreds of other attacks on government officials by traffickers, who murder those they cannot bribe. The strategy is summed up in the phrase *plomo o plata*, lead or silver, bullets or money.

In addition to its obvious negative impact on Latin American political systems, drug trafficking brings some liabilities for the economies as well. Inflation frequently accompanies the influx of coca dollars. Coca cultivation diverts land and labor from food crops and thus increases dependence on foreign imports. And the slash-and-burn cultivation techniques devastate tropical forests and erode future farmlands. Adding to the ecological damage are the chemicals used in cocaine refining.

... And Both Sides Benefit

If both North Americans and Latin Americans suffer from the illegal drug trade, both also reap its financial benefits. The benefits for the Andean producers are well-known. Cocaine trafficking is a major employer in a region of high unemployment. In the "White Triangle" of Bolivia, Peru and Colombia an estimated one million people, including farmers and laborers, are engaged in growing coca leaves and processing and exporting cocaine products. The earnings from this industry provide a vital source of foreign currency. Repatriated drug dollars "reactivated" the Colombian economy in 1987, according to the Colombian controller-general. A report by Bolivia's Chamber of Deputies says that cocaine exports were equal in value to that impoverished country's gross national product in 1985. Peru earns at least a third of its hard currency from growing coca and exporting pasta básica to Colombia, and the percentage rises as the Peruvian

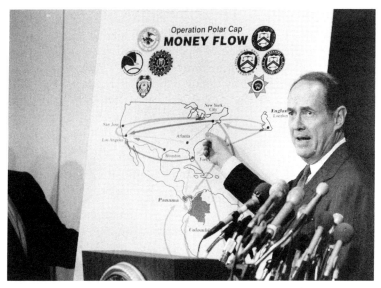

Attorney General Dick Thornburgh explaining an international money-laundering operation that shipped more than $1 billion a year in drug profits to a Colombian cartel.

economy slides deeper into depression. On days when the dollar shot up suddenly on the Lima black market in 1988, the joke was that the demand for dollars surpassed supply because the plane full of narcodollars hadn't arrived "from the mountain," or from the cocaine-trafficking Upper Huallaga Valley.

Whatever is earned from cocaine in South America, much more is earned in the United States. The U.S. market is the big jackpot in the smuggling game. A *Wall Street Journal* analyst conservatively estimated U.S. wholesale cocaine revenues in 1984 at $15 billion. This money is multiplied many times as cocaine is moved from the top of the trafficking pyramid down to the buyer on a U.S. city street. *The Tampa Tribune* reported that drugs have become an industry that earns Florida an estimated $6 billion annually, more than agriculture and second only to tourism. So many drug dollars enter Florida that the Federal Reserve Bank in Miami accumulates more currency than any other branch in the country. Money laundering is such a thriving business in Miami that investigators say it sustains large numbers of lawyers, bankers, accountants and brokers. It has even given rise to a new professional: drug couriers called "smurfs," who go from bank to bank buying cashier's checks. But Miami isn't the only place in the United States with a strong drug economy. Whole counties on the U.S.-Mexican border depend on drug smuggling to survive. One poor Oklahoma town was revived with drug dollars—and corrupted in the process. California's Humbolt County has lived on its marijuana crop for years. The hemisphere's illegal drug trade is truly a joint venture.

4

The Search for a Strategy

Looking back over the 20 years that have passed since Operation Intercept attempted to block the flow of Mexican marijuana, Washington can claim some successes for its antidrug policies in Latin America. Supported by more than $95 million in U.S. aid, Mexico carried out a marijuana and opium poppy eradication effort that did serious damage to the country's drug trade in the 1970s. Bowing to U.S. pressure, Colombian President Turbay signed an extradition treaty in 1979 and militarized the marijuana-trafficking Guajira Peninsula. Threatened with the loss of U.S. foreign aid, the Bolivian government set up a voluntary coca-eradication program that wiped out 2,570 acres in 1987 and early 1988. Do these short-term successes point toward a long-term victory over Latin American drug trafficking? The evidence suggests not. In fact, these cases point toward certain defeat. In Mexico, farmers used improved techniques of landscaping, fertilizing, irrigating and concealing their crops to produce bumper harvests of marijuana plants and opium poppies beginning in

1981. These new methods make eradication more costly and difficult. Mexico is once again this country's chief foreign supplier of heroin and marijuana. In Colombia, the military withdrew from the Guajira in fear of being corrupted by the traffickers, and the government set aside extradition after the Extraditables threatened the stability of the state. In Bolivia, while the government eradicates coca in some regions the peasants expand cultivation in others. This ebb-and-flow resulted in a net increase of 5,580 acres of new coca fields in little more than a year—1987 to early 1988.

As for the broader question of winning or losing the war on drugs, the answer is so obvious that there is no debate. The numbers speak for themselves: The amount of cocaine entering the country between 1984 and 1987 nearly quadrupled while its price went down as much as 40 percent, reaching a low of $80 a gram on the street. The only real achievements of U.S. drug diplomacy have been to increase friction with neighboring nations and to reinforce the stereotype of a heavy-handed Uncle Sam quick to bring his big stick down on Latin America.

Washington's errors began with the "war on drugs" metaphor. War is an image frequently used by politicians because it evokes strong sentiments against a common enemy. In an effort to mobilize mass support, recent U.S. Presidents have launched a "war on poverty," a "war on inflation" and a "war on drugs." The antidrug effort is the nearest of any of these to a real shoot-out between the forces of good (the police) and evil (the pushers), and it has passed into the popular imagination as an accurate picture of the problem. Thus the enormously complex issue of drug abuse and trafficking has been reduced to a matter of law enforcement. But, as Colombian President Barco argued in an editorial written for a U.S. newspaper, "if all that were required to stop drugs were the commitment and competence of law enforcement authorities in Colombia and the United States, we would have solved this deadly problem years ago." The problem persists, and the war on drugs is starting to look like what one expert calls the New Hundred Years' War. If the United States is to avoid endless conflict, politicians and the media will have to stop waging the war on drugs in speeches and headlines. The tough talk is producing no solutions. Another metaphor is needed.

An alternate image would be "drugs as plague." An *ABC News Special* in 1988 called drugs "A Plague Upon the Land." National leaders frequently refer to drugs as a scourge and an epidemic, but plagues and epidemics arise out of nature and descend upon humankind. The responsibility for these tragic events is not ours. Drug use is different. Users choose drugs. A baby born brain-damaged because its mother was a crack consumer certainly did not choose its fate, but nonetheless a choice was made—by the ignorant or indifferent mother. The U.S. drug problem is a conglomerate of millions of such decisions.

Drugs as Business

Until recently this element of choice was largely ignored, but a new generation of drug experts has put choice—the U.S. demand for drugs—at the center of their analytical model. The new thinking is based on economic rather than law-and-order logic. Laws still play a part, but they are the laws of supply and demand. The focus is on drugs as a business. This shift toward an economic model puts drugs in the proper perspective. It allows us to see that the United States should bankrupt the drug business by reducing demand.

Explored in think tanks, the economic model has shed new light on the obscure world of drug trafficking and produced new insights into U.S. policy failures. By reasoning back from drug seizures and street prices, economist Reuter has convincingly argued that interdiction can never decrease cocaine imports. No matter how many U.S. tax dollars are spent to seal the borders, cocaine will keep coming because there are so many methods of bringing drugs in and smuggling costs are such a small percentage of the final price of the product. If more drugs are seized, the traffickers will simply increase the amount sent, with only a negligible increase in price.

The supply-and-demand model of drug trafficking has moved out of the think tanks and into policymaking circles. In 1988 there

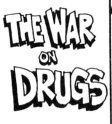
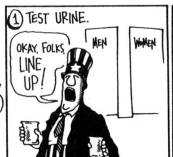
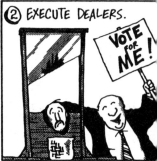

THE WAR ON DRUGS

① TEST URINE. OKAY, FOLKS, LINE UP! MEN WOMEN

② EXECUTE DEALERS. VOTE FOR ME!

was hardly a public official in Congress, the White House or the Justice Department who did not profess a determination to fight the supply of drugs by reducing demand. The Reagan Administration translated the supply-and-demand model into a policy of "get the users." Congress cooperated by passing a drug bill that imposed harsh penalties on users of even small amounts of marijuana.

Individual Rights Versus U.S. Drug Enforcement

Zero tolerance, critics claim, is doomed because demand cannot be repressed. Illicit drugs have been so persistently popular in the United States during this century that one big-city police chief calls the fight against them "one long glorious failure." Millions of U.S. citizens like drugs. Why they like drugs is another question. The answer may have something to do with the belief in the right to "the pursuit of happiness." Or perhaps the explanation can be found in what philosopher William James called the "moral weightlessness" of modern times. Whatever the reason, drugs, including alcohol and tobacco, are thoroughly woven into U.S. life. The government would have to rip apart the social fabric to extract illicit drug use from the U.S. national culture.

Some lawmakers are willing to take extreme measures to end the drug problem. Among the proposed amendments to the 1988 drug bill were the following provisions: permit police to make "good faith" drug searches without warrants; cut off Federal

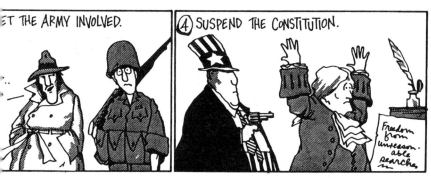

funds from companies that fail to ensure a "drug-free workplace," thus encouraging employers to spy on employees; and execute traffickers whether or not they had been involved in murders. Civil libertarians objected to these proposals as infringements on the Constitution, and they were removed from the final bill, but there is no guarantee they will not become law in the future. As public pressure builds to do something about drugs, politicians become more willing to compromise civil liberties. Drugs are a simmering social issue that can boil over into political demagoguery.

In the debate over individual rights versus drug enforcement, the question of drug testing occupies center stage. The spectrum of opinion on this issue stretches from those who believe with former President Reagan that testing should be carried out randomly at workplaces everywhere to those who consider mandatory urinalysis not only expensive and unreliable but an unacceptable invasion of privacy. In the two cases to reach the U.S. Supreme Court so far, justices ruled that railroad workers and U.S. Customs Service employees could be tested. The two cases raise different issues. Even staunch supporters of civil liberties can see an argument for testing transport workers as a matter of protecting the safety of the public, but public safety is not an issue for Customs Service workers. In his dissenting opinion, Justice Antonin Scalia called the Customs Service's random testing an "immolation of privacy and human dignity in symbolic opposition to drug use." The Customs Service decision has caused critics to accuse the court of making drug policy rather than defending the Constitution. Aside from the constitutional issues involved, testing seems unnecessary. After analyzing the urine samples of 2,100 of its employees, the Customs Service found only one with any trace of illegal drugs. These results hardly justify the Federal government's plan to expand its drug-testing program, which cost about $15 million in 1988. The challenge for the United States is to develop an antidrug policy that is both constitutional and within its budget.

Legalizing Drugs

Reflecting on past failures to repress drug demand and the high cost of continuing the same policies into the future, several scholars, newspaper columnists, police officers and top city officials have proposed legalization as an alternative. They argue that the problem is not the drugs but their illegality: antinarcotics laws make drug smuggling hugely profitable. Drug dealers would disappear just as bootleggers did after the end of Prohibition. With the stroke of a pen, legalization would unclog the courts, eliminate drug-gang violence in the inner cities and restore respect for the law by making it conform to practice. Some of the $8 billion spent by Federal, state and local governments to enforce drug laws could be funneled into antidrug education and treatment. These programs could also benefit from taxes on drugs like those levied on alcohol and tobacco.

In foreign relations, the legalization of drugs in the United States would pull out the props holding up the Latin American traffickers. Only its illegality explains why the product of the lowly coca bush costs 6,000 times more in New York City than the finest Colombian coffee. Legalization would topple this logic. The highly developed skills of the smugglers would have no value in an unrestricted market for cocaine. Legalization advocates argue that Latin America's underground empire would wither away, removing an obstacle in U.S.-Latin American relations.

This strong foreign policy argument must be tested against the impact legalization would have on U.S. society, particularly on the poverty-stricken inner cities. The middle class could save itself: those cocaine users with discipline could regulate their habits; those without could pay for drug treatment. But many observers are convinced that the desperate, uneducated poor are ill-equipped to resist crack cocaine sitting on a shelf in a corner store. DEA Chief John Lawn has warned that legalization would sign the death warrant for the ghetto. Lawn argues that the problem is not the laws, but the drugs themselves. He has a case when it comes to cocaine, a dangerously "reinforcing" drug which may be the most psychologically addictive substance in common use. Crack carries its users to an instant euphoria followed by a deep depression that can be lifted by more crack.

But Lawn's warning doesn't apply to marijuana. After 20 years of scientific studies there is convincing evidence that marijuana is not addictive and poses a health hazard no greater than tobacco. In 1988 the DEA's chief administrative law judge called marijuana "one of the safest therapeutically active substances known to man." Such statements give impetus to the argument that marijuana should be legalized. Opponents of marijuana legalization say it would increase the use of the drug, and some of the new marijuana users would eventually become cocaine and heroin users. Legalization advocates counter with the argument that there is nothing inherent in marijuana to create a need for harder drugs. If there is a link, proponents say, it is not the marijuana itself but the marijuana pusher. The pusher is a mobile market for all the drugs that cannot be purchased legally, from marijuana to heroin. The legalization of marijuana would separate it from the illegal market and thus diminish contact between marijuana consumers and hard-drug pushers. The experience of the Netherlands shows that the creation of a separate, legal market for marijuana can actually reduce heroin use.

The legalization of marijuana, some proponents argue, would also give the government new credibility as it attempts to educate the public about cocaine. The U.S. Surgeon General's successful campaign against cigarette smoking has shown that education is the most cost-effective way to change health-damaging behavior. This lesson could be applied to the drug problem. Drug use is a choice. Government can educate effectively about the consequences of that choice. Critics of the government's efforts to curb drugs claim that the government's information about narcotics has been so moralistic and so factually incorrect that users have rejected all warnings and experimented with any drug, no matter how dangerous. A government mature enough to put aside its alarmism about marijuana should be able to speak calmly and wisely about the real effects of cocaine. Funding for this anticocaine education effort could come from the former budget for marijuana repression. In 1987 the Federal government budgeted $3.8 million for eradication alone. That is more than the $3.5 million allocated in 1989 to the office of the new "drug czar," former Secretary of Education William Bennett.

A New Drug Diplomacy?

Although his funds are few and his statutory authority is limited, Bennett occupies a position with enough power and influence to reorient the U.S. antidrug effort from a "war" on drug suppliers to an educational campaign aimed at cutting drug demand and bankrupting the drug business. To do this Bennett would have to argue down those who see law enforcement as the answer. This pressure, which surges out of a frustrated population, has already pushed an unwilling Pentagon into drug interdiction. In 1988 Congress ordered the Department of Defense to play a greater role in narcotics interdiction by creating a drug intelligence network; providing support services to civilian agencies; and deploying the National Guard against trafficking. The Pentagon fears that soldiers will be corrupted by traffickers and that the military will become a scapegoat for the failures of U.S. drug policy. A more fundamental criticism is made by RAND economist Reuter. He says that the armed forces bring few relevant assets to the interdiction effort. For example, deploying high-tech military hardware is of little use if cocaine does not show up on radar screens. Military interdiction will only encourage smugglers to use commercial transport, as opposed to private planes, boats and trucks.

Given that the U.S. public wants antidrug enforcement to

continue, national leaders should try to scale down short-run expectations and set as a goal not winning a war but deflating the cocaine trade to manageable proportions. The Medellín cartel promoted U.S. drug consumption by turning random drug smuggling into an organized industry that cranked out cheap cocaine for millions of consumers. The most the United States can do is to push the drug business out of the mass market and back into the underground. This will be costly and difficult. One approach would be for law enforcers to tailor their efforts to the drugs-as-business pattern by using more intelligence and less force. Instead of kicking down doors, antidrug agents would spend more time chasing paper trails and doing Securities and Exchange Commission-style investigations. Only good intelligence work can tell the Customs Service which of the 7 million cargo containers entering the country every year contain illicit drugs. Intelligence work is difficult in drug-producing countries, where the power of drug dollars is great and U.S. investigators are hampered by their inexperience abroad. This is one argument for the DEA to shrink the number of its overseas agents and to rely more on carefully chosen and well-rewarded foreign agents and allies. Instead of organizing assaults on jungle cocaine laboratories in Peru and Bolivia, DEA personnel could put first priority on U.S. money laundering and other drug-related, white-collar crimes at home. This would encourage Latin America to fight drugs by emphasizing that the United States no longer considers drug trafficking some other nation's problem.

In acknowledging its role as the world's biggest consumer of illicit drugs, the United States has moved away from a strictly bilateral approach to drug diplomacy. Washington now says the drug fight must go multinational. In April 1988 Attorney General Meese proposed to Colombian President Barco that a multinational police force be deployed against the Medellín cocaine cartel. Colombia ignored the proposal and Bolivia flatly rejected it, but the proposal took shape in another form. The following August the DEA launched a series of joint operations in Latin America under the auspices of a 30-nation group called the International Drug Enforcement Conference. Multinational police operations were matched by an aggressive diplomatic effort. The State Department began lobbying international organizations and Western governments for greater cooperation in combating the Latin American traffickers.

The renewed U.S. willingness to work within world forums departed from previous Reagan Administration policy, offering evidence that the Administration was so alarmed by the drug danger that it was willing to reconsider its unbending commitment to independent foreign policy action. Latin American leaders had been seeking such a policy shift for some time. As Central America developed its own peace plan, and as Washington suffered foreign-policy defeats in Panama and Haiti, Latin America became impatient with any pretensions of U.S. hegemony in the hemisphere. The Bush Administration says it is sensitive to Latin America's new mood, but only time will tell if the United States can chart a successful antidrug policy in the hemisphere's changed diplomatic environment.

A truly multinational antidrug effort is likely to run into resistance within Washington itself. The DEA is dubious about working with governments in drug-producing countries, where corrupt leaders might tell traffickers about antidrug activities and thus put the lives of U.S. lawmen in danger. A case in point is the 1985 murder of DEA agent Enrique Camarena by traffickers allegedly protected by Mexican officials. If the DEA is suspicious of foreign governments, it also has reservations about its own. Agents complain about U.S. government priorities that put domestic politics and foreign policy concerns above fighting drugs. For example, the United States passed up a chance to capture top traffickers Jorge and Fabio Ochoa because the State Department feared their arrest would set off political disturbances in Colombia, according to a *Newsweek* report. Internal conflicts are constant because some three dozen different Federal offices are involved in Washington's antidrug effort. The ongoing interagency turf battles inside the U.S. government underscore the difficulty of uniting several governments in an antidrug alliance. Countries may hammer out a common program, but putting it into practice will be another matter. And then there is the question of money. How much will each member nation pay to sustain the joint antidrug effort? Recent history suggests that Washington does not want to bear a big part of the burden. Although the United States gives lip service to a multinational drug battle, words have not been backed up with large amounts of dollars. In 1988 the United States, the world's biggest consumer of illegal drugs, paid only 5 percent of the $60 million budget of the UN Fund for Drug Abuse Control.

5

Drugs or Development?

It is not enough for the United States to give up its gunboat diplomacy and adopt a more neighborly approach to the hemispheric drug problem. The rise of Latin America's drug industry parallels the decline of its national economies. Every year the region becomes more dependent on drug dollars. If the United States wants Latin America to kick the drug habit, Washington will have to offer more than moral support. In the final analysis any effort to bankrupt the drug business must be a coordinated campaign for economic development.

Burdened by a $420 billion foreign debt, Latin America wallows in its worst depression since the 1930s. Unemployment is at a record high. Average per capita income has dropped to its 1978 level, and in some countries living standards have slipped back two decades. The illicit drug industry keeps faltering economies from failing completely. As other sources of income decrease, trafficking in marijuana, cocaine and heroin increases. Although cause and effect cannot always be proven, correlation is undeniable in the case of Mexico. The 1982 "Mexican weekend" that heralded the country's debt crisis was followed immediately by a surge in illicit drug exports to the United States. Potent Mexican "black tar" heroin began pouring across the border, causing a sharp rise in heroin-related hospital emergencies in almost all western and southwestern U.S. cities since 1983. Mexican marijuana, which had been nearly eradicated in the 1970s, now tops the list of U.S. imports of that drug. Cocaine trafficking, a rarity before the economic crisis, has become big business. In October 1988 the Mexican army discovered 11,280 pounds of the drug hidden in caves not far from the Rio Grande.

Bolivia is another case study in the relationship between the collapse of a debt-burdened national economy and the rise of its drug business. In the first half of the 1970s Bolivia achieved an impressive economic growth rate of 6 percent a year, thanks to large foreign loans negotiated in expectation of the continued success of Bolivian metal exports, especially tin. The first sign of what was to come appeared in mid-decade when the world demand for cotton dropped and Bolivian agro-industrialists started exporting cocaine instead. Then tin prices took a dive in 1980, and Bolivia was forced to pay an ever-increasing percentage of its reduced export earnings to service the foreign debt. By 1981 Bolivia's debt problem had caused an economic crisis that spread over the whole country, pushing impoverished peasants and unemployed workers to cultivate coca. The final collapse came with the 1985 crash in the world market for tin, which lost half of its value in a single month. Former tin miners streamed into the coca-growing regions. Today Bolivia is a virtual *cocalandia*.

The rest of Latin America and the Caribbean have followed in the footsteps of Mexico and Bolivia. Venezuela, a big-borrowing member of the Organization of Petroleum Exporting Countries (OPEC) hit hard by the drop in world petroleum prices, has become an important bridge for Colombian cocaine. Another bridge country is economically stagnant Argentina, which has Latin America's third largest debt. In 1987 Argentine authorities seized more than half a ton of cocaine, compared with just 26 pounds three years before. Paraguay, long a major marijuana producer, is now a route to Europe for Bolivian cocaine. Jamaica and Belize are also marijuana-producers-turned-cocaine-traffickers. Haiti is a major cocaine transshipment point, and Ecuador, Honduras and Trinidad and Tobago are coming on-line. Brazil is both the Third World's biggest debtor and South America's only nation with an industrial base large enough to produce the chemical solvents needed for cocaine refining. Brazil looms as the coming giant in the drug industry.

The 'De-development' Decade

The correlation between debt and drugs is accompanied by another parallel relationship. The rise of the Latin American drug industry coincided with a decline in U.S. concern about economic growth in the region. For most of the post-World War II period Washington was engaged with Latin America in a development project of one kind or another, but the Reagan Administration disengaged from Latin America's most critical development issue, the foreign debt. While the debt burden pushed Latin America further into poverty, the Administration kept its distance from the crisis. The Administration's one substantial policy initiative was the Baker Plan, a moral appeal to U.S. banks to lend $20 billion to the 17 biggest debtor nations in the Third World, provided they adopt free-market economic policies. U.S. bankers resisted the plan, and the Administration didn't push the issue. Meanwhile interest payments siphoned off $25 billion a year that might have gone into economic development. Latin America looks back on the 1980s as a decade of de-development.

Latin America's economic crisis is not an abstract issue that concerns only economists. It affects directly the peasant farmers who are the foundation of the drug empire. More and more coca-growing peasants realize that their crop enslaves rather than serves humankind, but they see no alternate livelihood. Their economic prospects have never been good. Now they are terrible. "I don't know what we'd do without coca," one peasant told an Associated Press reporter in Bolivia. "What else is there?" What else, indeed. Bolivia has laid off 20,000 tin miners. They can stay in decaying company towns and survive on one meal a day of bread, bean leaves and potato peelings, or they can migrate to the Chapare region and grow coca. Faced with these choices, Bolivian tin miners find it very hard to "just say no" to coca.

The United States has undercut the alternatives to coca cultivation by raising nontariff barriers that impede imports from Latin America. In 1965 the United States had nontariff barriers against 27 percent of commodity imports. By 1986 more than half the imports to the United States were thus affected, but the illegal trade in drugs remained unrestricted. A direct cause-and-effect connection between rising U.S. restrictions on legitimate trade and the rise of trade in illicit drugs can be established in the case of marijuana cultivation in Belize. Washington set out to help Belize and other Caribbean countries through the Caribbean Basin Initiative (CBI), the Reagan Administration's one foray into the development field. But the CBI was hamstrung by reduced U.S. sugar quotas required by a U.S. farm bill that threw 100,000 Caribbean laborers out of work. As Congress repeatedly cut the amount of sugar Belize could sell to the United States, sugar farmers started growing marijuana. The trend was so obvious that early on the wife of one Belize sugar executive wrote First Lady Nancy Reagan a letter warning of an impending setback in the war on drugs. The message did not get through to policymakers in Washington. Belize became a major marijuana exporter. A similar shift is occurring in other Caribbean Basin countries. The irony is that while U.S. policy pushes Caribbean sugar farmers into marijuana, U.S. agricultural experts try to persuade coca-growing peasants in Bolivia and Peru to cultivate other crops.

Crop substitution offers the only hope of a supply-side solution to the drug problem, but exisiting programs are either so limited in scope and funds or so ineptly implemented that they can never wean Latin America from drug dependence. An example of a successful but underfunded project is a UN program that trades municipal improvements such as road construction and water pipelines for voluntary coca eradication by villagers in Colombia's Cauca Valley. As a result, cocaine production, drug-related violence and basuco addiction in the area are down. The former

65

head of Colombia's antinarcotics police believes the Cauca Valley project should be developed on a large scale, but that would require a much bigger budget than the $2.8 million provided by the UN and the matching funds from Colombian agencies.

An International Effort

In carrying out surgical strikes against drug trafficking the United States has not paid enough attention to Latin America's long-standing objections to interference by Uncle Sam. A successful crop substitution program would have to factor in Latin America's sensitivity about its sovereignty. This could be done by making crop substitution a multinational effort. The United States could enter into an alliance with other wealthy countries to fund a large-scale program. The UN Fund for Drug Abuse Control is presently supported by the United States, Britain, Canada, Italy and Saudi Arabia, and it could be expanded to oversee Latin America's transition from coca to other crops.

However it is administered, a Latin American crop substitution program would have to purchase entire harvests of both coca and the substitute crops for the number of years it would require to coax peasants out of one livelihood and into another. Over time the ratio of crops would shift away from coca and toward its alternatives. In the first year the international purchasing agency would buy up the entire coca harvest and destroy it, while in the last year of the program the agency would buy nothing but the substitute crops. An example of how this might work in practice is the UN program in the Cauca Valley, where coffee and avocado plants are planted around coca shrubs, eventually depriving the coca of light and killing it.

Any attempt to eliminate coca cultivation is a campaign to reorient the economies of whole countries and is thus costly by definition. The purchase of the coca crop would not be the largest item in the budget. Peasants earn so little from the sale of their coca leaves that 1988's entire harvest, estimated at between 97,000 and 124,000 metric tons, probably could have been bought for less than $2 billion. The big money is not coca but the infrastructure required to get alternative crops to market. The

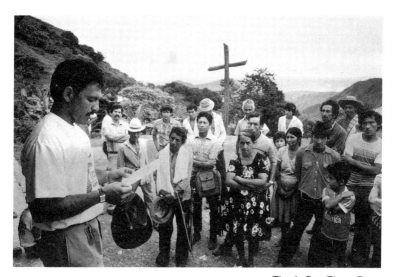

Coca growers in Cauca, Colombia, listening as a local official explains how the UN Coca Substitution Program works.

traffickers' clandestine landing strips in remote rural regions will not be open for legitimate products. The cost of constructing marketing mechanisms in Peru alone could be as much as $2 billion, according to Inter-American Dialogue, a Washington-based think tank.

It is appropriate that a crop-substitution agency invest in infrastructure because any effective antidrug effort must be accompanied by a global program of debt relief and economic development for Latin America. Only a comprehensive policy on the scale of the $13 billion Marshall Plan for European reconstruction after World War II can provide Latin America with a viable alternative to drug dependency. Before the drug prop can be pulled away, the United States and other drug-consuming countries will have to put something in its place.

Latin America recognizes that the responsibility for its future does not fall upon the United States. There is a new mood of self-reliance south of the border, as seen in the Contadora peace plan for Central America drafted by Colombia, Mexico, Panama and Venezuela and the Group of Eight (the Contadora countries plus Argentina, Brazil, Peru and Uruguay) meetings on the debt burden. But any realistic appraisal of Latin America's economic resources must conclude that the region cannot simply "go it alone." Latin America needs economic aid. The U.S. Congress is unlikely to expand aid for Latin America unless voters are convinced there is no alternative. Opinionmakers can rally voters around the antidrug banner and build an alliance that would attack not only drug trafficking but other hemispheric problems that can only be solved through joint efforts, such as immigration, ecology and the debt, which reduces Latin America's capacity to buy U.S. products. The alarming issue of drug abuse can be used to mobilize support for the less-headline-grabbing question of economic interdependence and Latin American development. What is needed is for Washington to make the connection between the crack sold on U.S. streets and the economic desperation of coca-growing peasants. The "cocaine connection" could pull this country into a new, more productive era in U.S.-Latin American relations. In 1988 the United States moved away from placing the blame for its drug habit on Latin America. That opened a door to a new hemispheric relationship. Now is the time for Washington to step forward and unite with Latin America in mutual cooperation against the common enemy, drugs.

Talking It Over

A Note for Students and Discussion Groups

This issue of the HEADLINE SERIES, like its predecessors, is published for every serious reader, specialized or not, who takes an interest in the subject. Many of our readers will be in classrooms, seminars or community discussion groups. Particularly with them in mind, we present below some discussion questions—suggested as a starting point only—and references for further reading.

Discussion Questions

The Pentagon wants to stay out of the fight against drug trafficking. Why? Shouldn't military technology such as radar be deployed in the interdiction of drugs? Assess the effectiveness of interdiction as an antidrug policy.

What does the author mean by the statement that "our errors began with the 'war on drugs' metaphor"? How do word pictures influence the way we think about things? What would be a better image than war for describing a policy to combat the illegal drug problem?

The author argues that the United States and Latin America are now both involved in the different aspects of the drug trade, from cultivation to money laundering and from health problems to police corruption. Is your community part of the "joint venture" of drugs?

Imagine that you are a Bolivian tin miner who has just lost his job. What would you do? Would you migrate to the Chaparé region and grow coca? Would you go to the U.S. embassy and ask for a visa to emigrate to the United States?

Has Colombia done enough to fight drugs? If Colombian police catch a major trafficker, should the United States seek his extradition? How does drug trafficking threaten democracy in Colombia? in the United States?

The U.S. State Department believes that the forced eradication of South American coca plantations can significantly reduce cocaine consumption in the United States. Do you agree? What are the social and political consequences of the U.S. coca eradication project in Peru's Upper Huallaga Valley? What is the environmental impact of eradication? of coca cultivation?

Does the drug industry contribute to the economic development of Latin America or is it just a stopgap measure that keeps economies from failing but does not contribute to the growth of their economic bases?

READING LIST

The Americas in 1989: Consensus for Action. Queenstown, Md., Inter-American Dialogue of The Aspen Institute, 1989. A succinct analysis of the Latin American crisis and what to do about it. Includes recommendations on drug trafficking.

Bagley, Bruce Michael, "Colombia and the War on Drugs." *Foreign Affairs,* Fall 1988. The rise of the illicit drug industry in Colombia and the U.S. response.

———, "The New Hundred Years War? U.S. National Security and the War on Drugs in Latin America." *Journal of Interamerican Studies and World Affairs,* Spring 1988. A review of failed U.S. policies and a summary of future options.

Collett, Merrill, "The Myth of the 'Narco-Guerrillas.'" *The Nation,* August 13/20, 1988. Claims of an alliance between drug traffickers and leftist insurgents are found unsupported by the facts.

Craig, Richard B., "Domestic Implications of Illicit Colombian Drug Production and Trafficking." *Journal of Interamerican Studies and World Affairs,* August 1983. One of the first scholarly accounts. Still useful for understanding the marijuana boom in Colombia.

Falco, Mathea, *Winning the Drug War: A National Strategy.* New York, Priority Press Publications for The Twentieth Century Fund, 1989. A former assistant secretary of state for international narcotics matters defines the drug problem and prescribes a strategy.

"The Great Drug Debate." *The Public Interest,* Summer, 1988. Articles by Ethan A. Nadelmann, the leading academic advocate of legalization, Peter Reuter, a RAND Corporation drug economist, and John Kaplan, a Stanford law school professor, focus on the issues involved.

Grinspoon, Lester, and Bakalar, James B., *Cocaine: A Drug and Its Social Evolution,* rev. ed. New York, Basic Books, 1985. A wealth of medical insight from two Harvard psychiatrists.

Hamowy, Ronald, ed., *Dealing With Drugs.* San Francisco, Calif., Pacific Research Institute for Public Policy, 1988. Libertarians argue that politicians have used the drug issue to serve their own agendas.

International Narcotics Control Strategy Report. U.S. Department of State, Bureau of International Narcotics Matters. Washington, D.C., U.S. Government Printing Office, 1988. The annual report prepared for Congress as part of the drug certification process.

McCoy, Alfred, *The Politics of Heroin in Southeast Asia.* New York, Harper & Row, 1972. The authoritative account of how CIA operations against communism in Asia created the largest single source of heroin for the U.S. market.

Pacini, Deborah, and Franquemont, Christine, eds., *Coca and Cocaine: Effects on People and Policy in Latin America.* Peterborough, N.H., Cultural Survival, 1986. The view from the grass roots by academic experts with extensive field experience in South America.

Shannon, Elaine, *Desperados.* New York, Viking, 1988. A journalistic account of marijuana in Mexico that reflects the DEA's defense of its policies.

Stone, Robert, "A Higher Horror of the Whiteness." *Harper's Magazine,* December 1987. A distinguished novelist looks at cocaine and the U.S. national character.

U.S. Postal Service

STATEMENT OF OWNERSHIP, MANAGEMENT AND CIRCULATION
Required by 39 U.S.C. 3685)

1A. Title of Publication	1B. PUBLICATION NO.	2. Date of Filing
Headline Series	0 0 1 7 8 7 8 0	9/20/89

3. Frequency of Issue	3A. No. of Issues Published Annually	3B. Annual Subscription Price
Quarterly: Winter, Spring, Summer, Fall	Four	$15.00

4. Complete Mailing Address of Known Office of Publication *(Street, City, County, State and ZIP+4 Code) (Not printers)*

Foreign Policy Association, 729 Seventh Avenue, NY, NY, 10019

5. Complete Mailing Address of the Headquarters of General Business Offices of the Publisher *(Not printer)*

same as above

6. Full Names and Complete Mailing Address of Publisher, Editor, and Managing Editor *(This item MUST NOT be blank)*

Publisher *(Name and Complete Mailing Address)*

Foreign Policy Association, 729 Seventh Avenue   NY, NY   10019

Editor *(Name and Complete Mailing Address)*

Nancy Hoepli, same as above

Managing Editor *(Name and Complete Mailing Address)*

n/a

7. Owner *(If owned by a corporation, its name and address must be stated and also immediately thereunder the names and addresses of stockholders owning or holding 1 percent or more of total amount of stock. If not owned by a corporation, the names and addresses of the individual owners must be given. If owned by a partnership or other unincorporated firm, its name and address, as well as that of each individual must be given. If the publication is published by a nonprofit organization, its name and address must be stated.) (Item must be completed.)*

Full Name	Complete Mailing Address
Foreign Policy Association	729 Seventh Avenue, NY, NY, 10019

8. Known Bondholders, Mortgagees, and Other Security Holders Owning or Holding 1 Percent or More of Total Amount of Bonds, Mortgages or Other Securities *(If there are none, so state)*

Full Name	Complete Mailing Address
n/a	n/a

9. For Completion by Nonprofit Organizations Authorized to Mail at Special Rates *(DMM Section 423.12 only)*
The purpose, function, and nonprofit status of this organization and the exempt status for Federal income tax purposes *(Check one)*

(1) [X] Has Not Changed During Preceding 12 Months	(2) [ ] Has Changed During Preceding 12 Months	*(If changed, publisher must submit explanation of change with this statement.)*

10. Extent and Nature of Circulation *(See instructions on reverse side)*	Average No. Copies Each Issue During Preceding 12 Months	Actual No. Copies of Single Issue Published Nearest to Filing Date
A. Total No. Copies *(Net Press Run)*	11,227	11,450
B. Paid and/or Requested Circulation 1. Sales through dealers and carriers, street vendors and counter sales	3,904	1,017
2. Mail Subscription *(Paid and/or requested)*	3,354	3,658
C. Total Paid and/or Requested Circulation *(Sum or 10B1 and 10B2)*	7,258	4,675
D. Free Distribution by Mail, Carrier or Other Means Samples, Complimentary, and Other Free Copies	500	500
E. Total Distribution *(Sum of C and D)*	7,758	5,175
F. Copies Not Distributed 1. Office use, left over, unaccounted, spoiled after printing	3,469	6,275
2. Return from News Agents	-0-	-0-
G. TOTAL *(Sum of E, F1 and 2—should equal net press run shown in A)*	11,227	11,450

11. I certify that the statements made by me above are correct and complete	Signature and Title of Editor, Publisher, Business Manager, or Owner
	Dir., Finance & Admin. *Mark S. Callahan*

PS Form **3526**, Feb. 1989   *(See instructions on reverse)*